Y0-AAG-939

Monographs

of the Yale Center of Alcohol Studies

No. 3

Monographs of the Yale Center of Alcohol Studies

Under the editorship of Mark Keller

The Yale Center of Alcohol Studies is a section of the Yale University Laboratory of Applied Biodynamics. The Monographs in this series report the results of original research in any of the scientific disciplines, whether carried out at Yale or elsewhere.

No. 1. Alcohol and the Jews. A Cultural Study of Drinking and Sobriety. By CHARLES R. SNYDER. $5.00

No. 2. Revolving Door. A Study of the Chronic Police Case Inebriate. By DAVID J. PITTMAN and C. WAYNE GORDON. $4.00

No. 3. Alcohol in Italian Culture. Food and Wine in Relation to Sobriety among Italians and Italian Americans. By GIORGIO LOLLI, EMIDIO SERIANNI, GRACE M. GOLDER and PIERPAOLO LUZZATTO-FEGIZ. $4.00

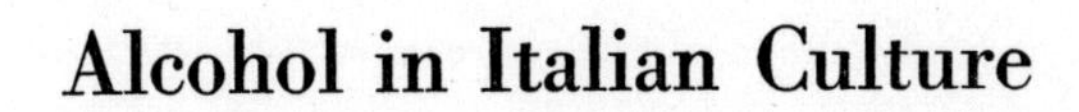

Alcohol in Italian Culture

Bibliographic Note

Some preliminary and part results of the studies reported here in Part I were published previously in the Quarterly Journal of Studies on Alcohol (Bibliography, references 13, 18, 19 and 20). The present Part I, however, is not a reprint of those reports but a new work.

Part II was published previously in the Quarterly Journal of Studies on Alcohol, Vol. 18, No. 3, pp. 355–381, 1957.

Alcohol in Italian Culture

Food and Wine in Relation to Sobriety among Italians and Italian Americans

BY

GIORGIO LOLLI, M.D.

EMIDIO SERIANNI, M.D.

GRACE M. GOLDER, R.N., M.A.

AND

PIERPAOLO LUZZATTO-FEGIZ, LL.D.

THE FREE PRESS
GLENCOE, ILLINOIS

PUBLICATIONS DIVISION:
YALE CENTER OF ALCOHOL STUDIES
NEW HAVEN, CONNECTICUT

Library of Congress catalog card number: 58-9167

MANUFACTURED IN THE UNITED STATES OF AMERICA BY
UNITED PRINTING SERVICES, INC.
NEW HAVEN, CONN.

Contents

List of Tables

Part I

Part II

Introduction

That alcoholism is a "problem," whether social or medical or both, is generally agreed. Less generally recognized is the fact that this problem requires systematic study, and that knowledge derived from disciplined inquiry can help to solve it. It must be admitted that there is a substantial body of popular opinion which holds that alcoholism does not merit the special attention of scientists. In this view, alcoholism is simply a byproduct of drinking alcoholic beverages and the solution of the problem is self-evident: universal total abstinence.

This latter viewpoint immediately points to drinking as a problem. And it might be supposed that drinking behavior, especially as some of its aspects are manifestly related to serious medical and social disorders, would be a focus of interest for a number of sciences. As a matter of fact, sociologists managed for a long time to ignore drinking as an area of potential investigation. Perhaps they had just as good reason for this avoidance as medical scientists had for their avoidance of alcoholism. But the time is past when any of the disciplines can ignore either drinking or alcoholism. The pages of such a periodical as the QUARTERLY JOURNAL OF STUDIES ON ALCOHOL demonstrate that in widening scientific circles the awareness is growing that both drinking and alcoholism are areas of vital and fruitful research. Perhaps this means that the bitter traditional opponents in the controversy about "alcohol," the "Wets" and the "Drys," can be seen in their proper perspective, as material for study, while their narrow theories are set aside and rational hypotheses are tested by disciplined methods. The present work reports an attempt along this line. Its particular concern is the possible relationship of a national drinking pattern to sobriety rather than alcoholism. Its ultimate basis is the perception that not just problem drinking but all drinking is the interest of science.

That drinking must precede alcoholism is obvious. Equally obvious, but not always sufficiently considered, is the fact that drinking is not necessarily followed by alcoholism. If the origin of alcoholism is ever to be understood, if the prevention of alcoholism—other than by the unlikely radical abolition of alcohol—is ever to be achieved, it will be necessary to gain fundamental understanding, among other things, of the real relationship not only between drinking and alcoholism, but also between drinking and other activities. What are the kinds of drinking patterns, the attitudes about drinking, the behaviors related to drinking, the amounts or rates of drinking, or perhaps the kinds or strengths of beverages, which are associated with the development of alcoholism? And what kinds of drinking patterns, attitudes, related behaviors, and so forth, are associated with sobriety?[1]

The last question may be painful to those who have perceived no more than the simple relationship: drinking→alcoholism. But it must be asked and answered, and in recent years an increasing number of investigators have launched upon studies related to this problem. For it was impossible not to notice that within the general society, plagued by a variety of alcohol-related problems, there were recognizable subgroups which seemed immune to them. First there are the Jews, and an extensive literature attests to the rarity of alcoholism among them. This fact has most recently been thoroughly documented by Snyder (30), who has demonstrated in his study that the freedom of the Jews from "alcohol pathologies" is in contrast to their extensive practice of drinking all sorts of alcoholic beverages. The Chinese in America, as Barnett (2) has shown, are another group free of alcoholism in spite of widespread drinking. And finally there are the Italians. In this group, the focus of the present study, it will be seen that the drinking of wine is almost universal. Yet among persons arrested for drunkenness (28) and among patients of alcoholism clinics (13), Italians are relatively scarce.

It seemed especially worth while to concentrate a substantial research effort on the Italian-American subgroup because of the possibility of conducting parallel studies among the Italians in the homeland. A large portion of the Americans of Italian descent are still little removed in terms of generation, time and cultural influence from their ancestors. The present research was therefore designed to take advantage of this situation.

First, a series of studies was undertaken as joint projects of the

[1] These questions do not substitute for others, equally pertinent, concerning the possible roles of personality, physiological, biochemical, constitutional, hereditary and perhaps still other factors; they are emphasized here in line with the specific focus of the present work. The full range of potential research on alcohol problems in the social sciences was outlined long ago by Bacon (1) and in other disciplines by Jellinek (6).

Yale Plan Clinic (a division of the Yale University Laboratory of Applied Biodynamics and Center of Alcohol Studies) of New Haven, Connecticut, and the Istituto di Alimentazione e Dietologia in Rome. Over-all responsibility for the projects was carried by Dr. Giorgio Lolli, then Medical Director of the Yale Plan Clinic. Dr. Emidio Serianni, Director of the Istituto di Alimentazione e Dietologia, was responsible for the planning and execution of the project in Italy. In various phases of the work they were aided in Italy by Claudia Balboni, M.D., Ferruccio Banissoni, M.D., Violetta Belcecchi Meschieri, M.A., Adriana Leproux, M.A., Aldo Mariani, M.D., Anna Muratori Traversa, M.D., Gabriella Pallone Gardini, M.A., Gloria Pepi, M.S., Clara Perri, B.A., Marcello Proja, M.D. and Carlo Traversa, M.D.; and in the United States by Edith Lisansky, Ph.D., Raymond G. McCarthy, M.A., M.Ed., Ruth Smith, B.A., Robert Straus, Ph.D., Mary Toner, R.N., M.A., and Bella Wu.

The methods and rationales of investigation will not be recited here, since they are detailed in the text. But it is necessary to explain the division of this report into two parts and the difference between the two separate samples studied in each major part.

One group of studies, reported here in Part I, was carried out in parallel samples of Italians in Italy and Americans of Italian extraction in New Haven.[2] Although there is reason to think, on the basis of experience, that these samples substantially resemble the larger Italian and Italian-American populations from which they were drawn, no claims to randomness or representativeness in the strict sampling sense can be made for them. The circumstances of the study did not allow more exact procedures in composing these samples. Nevertheless, consideration of the basic attitudes which underlie the drinking and other behaviors described in Parts I and II has given the investigators the very strong impression that the Part I samples tap what is essentially Italian. Indeed, similarities between first-generation Italian Americans and Italians in Italy are striking, and the changes which begin to manifest themselves in the second and third generations seem to rein-

[2] Some part results of the studies presented in Part I have been reported previously (13, 18, 19, 20), but the present work is a new summarization, not a reprint of those preliminary statements. Part II, however, has been published previously substantially in its present form in the QUARTERLY JOURNAL OF STUDIES ON ALCOHOL, Vol. 18, No. 3, pp. 355–381, September 1957.

force the similarity of the basic traits which go into the drinking and drinking-related behaviors. Thus, while it cannot be asserted that the facts elicited in Part I apply strictly to the two general populations sampled, it seems warranted to think that the samples are sufficiently representative to give a reasonable degree of validity to the findings.

In the case of the study reported in Part II, however, the situation is quite different. For this investigation a stratified sample of the adult population of Italy was used. The findings thus reliably describe certain behaviors of adult Italians in contemporary times. These findings, and those of Part I to the extent that they run parallel, constitute a contribution to the growing body of knowledge concerning those drinking and drinking-related behaviors and attitudes which do not lead to social pathologies but are associated rather with essential sobriety. This is, moreover, the second contribution to this category of knowledge arising from the broad interest of the Yale Center of Alcohol Studies in research on non-problem as well as problem drinking. The first, already mentioned, is the study of drinking in Jewish culture as recently described by Snyder (30).

Research is not undertaken in a vacuum, and research workers do not blindly go gathering odds and ends of facts. The present studies were undertaken with a definite problem in mind and within a definite frame of reference. The investigators believed, to begin with, that the drinking habits of Italians were closely interwoven with their dietary habits. Accordingly the research was organized so as to elicit information about drink and diet and their interrelation. It will be seen that the findings in both Parts I and II demonstrate the high importance of this relationship. If what has been learned thus far were to be summarized in a few words, it could be said that for Italians drinking is a part of eating, even a form of eating, for wine is a food; that to the extent that the descendants of Italians in America retain ancestral cultural traditions, they drink with the same attitudes and in the same ways; and that the set of attitudes which does not separate drink from food is at least partly responsible for the relative sobriety of Italian drinking. Other features of Italian culture have been pointed to —such as certain aspects of the early child-rearing complex—which may play a role in personality development conducive to the prevention of inebriety. But these features could not be sufficiently elucidated in the present studies to allow more than the formulation of suggestions and theories.

Whether and how this sort of information can be applied to the solution of the problem of inebriety where it exists remains to be seen. It is certain, however, that only through the steady accumulation, refinement, synthesis and objective interpretation of such knowledge will it become possible to achieve rational solutions to the problems of alcohol and alcoholism.

MARK KELLER

Part I

Drinking and Meals among Italians and Italian Americans

BY

Giorgio Lolli, M.D.

Emidio Serianni, M.D.

AND

Grace M. Golder, R.N., M.A.

Chapter 1

PROBLEM AND METHOD

INTRODUCTION

ONE of the most striking elements of the problem of alcoholism is the great variation in the incidence of this condition in different cultures and different nationality groups. For example, according to a World Health Organization estimate (8) the rate of alcoholism was approximately 3,950 per 100,000 adults in the United States, but only 500 per 100,000 in Italy. Interestingly, 25 per cent of the American cases but nearly all the Italian cases were classified as alcoholism with complications. The "complications" are mostly nutritional disorders.

The eight-fold difference in the frequency of alcoholism can hardly be attributed to a larger consumption of alcohol in the United States. The per capita use of alcohol is substantially larger in Italy (10).

A similar and equally startling difference is apparent from a review of the work of the Yale Plan Clinic at New Haven, Conn. Of the first 1,200 addictive drinkers who attended that clinic, only 40 (3 per cent) were of Italian extraction (18). This very low incidence of Italian alcoholics is particularly noteworthy since individuals of Italian extraction comprise more than 25 per cent of the total population of New Haven. It also appears significant that all of the 40 Italian-American alcoholics were not recent immigrants but second- or third-generation Americans, and that most of them were addicted to the use of distilled spirits.

It is a pressing necessity to discover explanations for these and similar variations—to cast some light on the factors which allow large segments of the world's population to consume alcoholic beverages, sometimes in considerable amounts, without experiencing noticeable difficulties with themselves and their environments, while other groups attempting to use these beverages are faced with serious problems.

Accordingly, the present investigation was undertaken on a group of Italians born and living in Italy—a group characterized by relative freedom from alcoholism—as well as on a group of

Americans of Italian extraction, both to be studied with identical techniques. It was hoped that this project might indicate at least some of the factors in the cultural environment of the Italians which, over the centuries, have served to protect them from the excessive or dangerous use of alcoholic beverages. Such a study, it was felt, might clarify some of the differences between addictive and non-addictive individuals, and perhaps help to isolate and identify some factors contributing to the causation of alcoholism.

Basically, this was designed as an investigation of nutritional patterns. Within the frame of the Italian culture—a term aptly defined by André Malraux as the "incarnation of a system of values" (23)—the tie between drinking and eating was obvious. Italians have apparently always viewed the use of wine as an integral part of their nutrition. Among Italian Americans, the connection between drinking and eating might be less obvious.[1] Nevertheless, it seemed evident that drinking habits are nutritional habits—and alcoholism, an extreme deviation of a drinking habit, is therefore an extreme deviation of a nutritional habit (16).

When such deviations are considered, whether they are expressed as alcoholism or overdrinking, or as obesity or overeating, it is clear that they cannot be adequately explained, prevented or controlled by purely medical approaches (16). These problems involve not only physiological and biochemical factors, but also the cultural background of an individual, his emotional make-up, and the impact of social pressures upon him. A great wealth of knowledge has been accumulated on the psychological and sociocultural aspects of sex, for example, but although nutrition as a biological process is more fundamental than sex, most of the psychological and sociocultural aspects of eating and drinking have been neglected by systematic students.

A second neglected area has been that concerned with the ingestion of liquids, alcoholic or nonalcoholic. With the exception of milk, the consumption of fluids by individuals or groups has been largely or entirely ignored. Most surveys or dietary studies have paid little or no attention to the use of alcoholic and nonalcoholic beverages, and there is practically no instance of a dietary study which included a careful inquiry on water. Yet water, though lack-

[1] For an earlier intensive study of the drinking practices of a small group of Italian Americans in New Haven see Williams and Straus (31).

ing any caloric value, must be considered as a vital nutritional element.

The present nutritional inquiry, therefore, was concerned with all components of the diet, solid and liquid, alcoholic and nonalcoholic. It was likewise concerned with psychological and sociocultural factors which may affect nutrition—factors ranging from the religious and political views of the subjects to their attitudes toward children, property and sex.

Although a considerable amount of information was obtained from the subjects participating in this research, the data in no case were sufficient to describe the total personalities of the subjects or to support any far-reaching conclusions on personality. Moreover, this was not to be a "cultural study," and did not attempt to define the characteristic traits of Italians in Italy or of Italian Americans in the United States.

Instead, major efforts were devoted to gathering information from the subjects in certain physiological, psychological and sociocultural areas, and correlating this information with the eating and drinking habits of the subjects. The results, presented in the following chapters, seem to cast light on some factors which may play a vital role in the prevention of alcoholism.

Methods[2]

At the outset of this investigation, it was accepted that the eating and drinking habits of an individual are determined by the same forces of heredity and environment which operate in all human behavior.

In the case of eating and drinking patterns, heredity plays a necessary although perhaps minor role which, at this stage of our scientific knowledge, cannot be adequately defined. On the other hand, certain relationships of the individual to his environment and certain factors in the development of his personality are more clearly understood. Through the application of widely accepted principles of dynamic psychology, it is possible to trace the development of those factors which ultimately contribute to the normal or deviant eating and drinking behavior of the adult.

[2] Dr. Milton Silverman was particularly helpful in the early stages of the planning of this project, in the evaluation of the gathered data and, finally, in the editorial work of preparing this monograph for publication.

At present, it appears that a psychodynamic, Freudian-inspired interpretation is the most satisfactory for analyzing those events which, starting with early infancy, lead to contemporary behavior. It encompasses all physiological, psychological, social, ethical and religious factors. It makes possible the adequate evaluation of the physiological events which affect normal or abnormal behavior of many kinds, including nutritional behavior.

In the light of this viewpoint, an attempt was made in this study to gather as much information as possible not merely on grams or cubic centimeters of food and beverage consumed, but also on the physiological, psychological and social attitudes of a group of individuals who were nutritionally within reasonable limits of normality.

Selection of Subjects

In developing the project,[3] efforts were made to include subjects whose origins stemmed from Northern, Central and Southern Italy. Consequently, in Italy, the metropolitan district of Rome was chosen as an area containing representatives of all sections of the country, and a group of subjects was selected and studied there. These comprised the group known as the Italians.

At the same time, individuals of Northern, Central or Southern Italian origin were studied in the United States in New Haven, Conn. All of them were residents of the city, and volunteered to cooperate with the Yale Plan Clinic in the research project as a result of information given to Italian clubs, social groups and social agencies having a large number of Italian clients on their lists, and to individual members of the Italian community. These are the first-, second- and third-generation subjects who will be referred to as Italian Americans.

Efforts were made to select the members of the two groups so they would be generally similar in age, sex, education, religion, economic status, and both physical and emotional health.

Each subject was interviewed by a member of the investigating staff before being accepted, so that he understood clearly what was expected of him.

Contact with each subject was maintained for periods varying from several weeks to several months. During this time, each one

[3] Detailed descriptions of the initiation of this project and portions of the findings have been published previously (13, 18, 19, 20) by Lolli, Serianni et al.

prepared a dietary record and underwent a sociological examination, a physical examination, a sugar tolerance test, and several psychological examinations.

The Dietary Diary

The core of this research project was the dietary diary. For years, such a diary—although its validity has occasionally been challenged—has been a useful tool in research on the nutritional status of individuals and groups. In addition, it was felt that the dietary diary could not only supply useful information on the nutritional habits of the individual but would also serve as a simple and useful opening wedge into his emotional life.

There are large segments of the population which resent most vigorously any intimation that the emotional life of the individual revolves to a large extent around the adequacy or inadequacy of his sexual attitudes. With such people, inquiries centered around eating and drinking habits and nutritional attitudes offer better chances of being accepted without hostility or prejudice, and can smoothly open the way to further investigation.

In addition, interviews centered on nutritional habits advantageously focus the attention of the investigator and the subject on events which occurred at the very dawn of psychological life—events linked with the so-called oral stage of psychological development. Thus, the establishment of rapport on a "nutritional" basis provides a contact on this important early level. The establishment of such a contact calls for great skill on the part of the interviewer, but it is highly rewarding. As one dividend from this study, it was found that through nutritional inquiries, psychologically trained personnel may contribute significantly and with a minimum of effort to mental hygiene and the prevention of mental illness.

To each candidate for participation, both in Italy and in the United States, the project was carefully interpreted for what it really was: an inquiry centered on the nutritional habits of individuals of Italian extraction in this country and of Italians in Italy. The inquiry, it was emphasized, had many goals—particularly a clarification of those factors which, to a certain extent, protect the Italian population from the problems of excessive drinking of alcohol. The interviewers, however, avoided giving the impression that the goal of the project might be to prove any superiority of the Italians or of the Italian Americans.

The candidates were likewise told that little is known of what comprises the normal person's nutritional pattern. Although average values are available concerning proteins, fats, carbohydrates, vitamins and minerals, there is little information on the timing of food ingestion, the setting, the company, the type of conversation at the dinner table, emotions connected with eating or not eating, reasons why some items of food are liked and why some are repulsive, and so on.

Essentially all candidates showed keen interest in these explanations, and the majority of those interviewed in Italy and all those interviewed in this country agreed to participate in the project.

At a special meeting with each subject, full instructions were presented on the dietary diary and ample time was provided to answer any questions which he might present.

The diary itself consisted of seven simple mimeographed sheets, one for each day of a week. The one-week period was selected since there are reasons to believe that the average housewife exhausts her culinary repertoire during that period (25) and accordingly a week's record would give a general idea of the foods and beverages usually ingested by each subject. The record weeks were spread approximately equally over the seasons of the year.

Each sheet was identified only by a case number. The subjects were not required to identify their reports with their names, since it was felt that in some cases the ingestion of food may be connected with inhibitions and feelings as strong as those linked with sexual activity.

The diary sheet was divided into two columns, one for the listing of all solid foods and the other for all liquid foods or beverages —including water. Immediately after each item was ingested, the time of ingestion was to be recorded, together with the quantity of the item in terms of cupfuls and spoonfuls. When mixed dishes were involved, the subject was instructed to list all ingredients. It was obvious that such measurements would be only approximations, but extensive studies have shown that these individual records are valuable in nutritional surveys, especially when an adequate number of subjects is included (25).

At the bottom of each page, ample space was left for the subject to record any occurrences of the day which might have affected his eating pattern or any other unusual events.

In case any question arose concerning the weight of some food item, the type of cooking involved, or any other facet of the inquiry, the subject was asked to telephone to the clinic for advice or information.

When the word "diet" was first mentioned to the subjects, it was apparent at once that many felt their diet was to be criticized, and most of them made more or less disparaging remarks about their own food habits. Accordingly, the subjects were told that the survey was not concerned with the nutritional adequacy of a diet, and that the interviewers would not judge whether the diets were "right" or "wrong." In the same way, this nonjudgmental attitude on the part of the interviewer presumably helped to overcome the unconscious tendency of the obese subject to omit some items from his records, and of the underweight subject to magnify his intake of food.

Each subject was told that practically all diets are more or less deficient in one or more nutrients, and that, once his diet had been calculated from the dietary diary, he would be able to ascertain by himself whether or not he fell below recommended standards.

It was decided at the outset of the project that no observers should be used to watch the subjects during their meals. Since inhibitions and blockings may exist in the area of hunger-linked emotions, and of all activities connected with food, it was felt that many individuals would resent supervision while eating. The mere presence of an observer could unconsciously distort the basic picture of the eating pattern. It appeared that a more truthful and accurate picture could be obtained by relying on the statements presented by the subjects themselves on their uses of food and on their attitudes and feelings linked with the ingestion of food.

Chapter 2

CHARACTERISTICS OF THE SAMPLE

As a first step, information was obtained from all subjects on their parents, and on their own heights, weights, marital status, religious attitudes and practices, languages spoken and understood, education, economic status and medical status.

The results of these preliminary investigations are presented in the following sections.

Sex and Age

A total of 498 men and women—247 Italians and 251 first-, second- and third-generation Italian Americans—served as the subjects in the investigation.

In this sample, attempts were made to have an adequate representation of subjects in different age groups. As shown in Table 1, most were between the ages of 20 and 60.

Region of Origin

The Italian subjects were almost evenly divided by regional origin among the three major divisions of the country—79 from Northern Italy, 80 from Central Italy and 88 from Southern Italy. Among the Italian Americans, a northern origin was reported for 87, and a central origin for 60, while 104 were of southern extraction. The preponderance of those of southern origin among the Italian Americans conforms to the fact that the majority of Italian immigrants in the eastern United States came from Southern Italy.

A total of 72 subjects were born in Italy and migrated to the United States. The age at which these first-generation Italian Americans arrived in this country is as follows: less than 10 years, 7 men and 14 women; 10–19, 12 men and 12 women; 20–29, 6 men and 12 women; 30–39, 3 men and 4 women; and over 40, 1 man. In one case this information was not obtained.

Parents of the Subjects

The fathers and mothers of all the Italian subjects were born in Italy. The country of birth of the parents of the Italian-American subjects is shown in Table 2. It can be seen that about 45 per

TABLE 1.—*Age and Sex of Subjects (in Per Cent)*

NOTE: In this and subsequent tables, data on the Italian-American group are subdivided under each sex by generations, identified by the column headings "1st" and "2d+3d." Data on second- and third-generation Italian Americans were combined because of insufficient differences to warrant separate tabulation. The few interesting differences are noted in the text.

ITALIANS				ITALIAN AMERICANS				
Male	*Female*	*Total*		*Male*		*Female*		*Total*
				1st	2d+3d	1st	2d+3d	
(*N*=*125*)	(*N*=*122*)	(*N*=*247*)		(*N*=*28*)	(*N*=*81*)	(*N*=*44*)	(*N*=*98*)	(*N*=*251*)
5	4	5	Under 20	0	10	0	7	6
17	16	17	20–24	0	21	5	11	12
32	17	25	25–29	7	15	2	24	15
19	16	18	30–34	11	21	9	17	16
11	16	14	35–39	4	20	18	15	16
5	8	6	40–44	0	9	14	11	10
6	8	7	45–49	18	2	9	7	7
2	7	4	50–54	7	1	9	2	4
2	6	3	55–59	25	1	14	1	6
2	2	2	60 and over	29	0	20	4	8
101	*100*	*101*	*Totals*	*101*	*100*	*100*	*99*	*100*

TABLE 2.—*Birthplace and Migration of Parents of Italian-American Subjects (in Per Cent)*

FATHER		MOTHER		ITALIAN AMERICANS				
				Male		*Female*		*Total*
Country of Birth	*Migrated to U.S.*	*Country of Birth*	*Migrated to U.S.*	1st (*N*=*28*)	2d+3d (*N*=*81*)	1st (*N*=*44*)	2d+3d (*N*=*98*)	(*N*=*251*)
U.S.	—	U.S.	—	0	10	2	10	7
Italy	Yes	Italy	Yes	43	69	43	78	65
Italy	Yes	U.S.	—	0	1	0	0	0
U.S.	—	Italy	Yes	0	16	0	11	10
Italy	No	Italy	No	46	4	45	0	14
Italy	No	Italy	Yes	7	0	0	0	1
Italy	Yes	Italy	No	4	0	5	0	1
No information		No information		0	0	5	1	1
Totals				*100*	*100*	*100*	*100*	*99*

cent of both the men and women among the first-generation subjects were born of parents who did not come to the United States.

The parents of all the Italian subjects were Italian citizens. Of the Italian Americans, as shown in Table 3, 75 per cent of the first-generation men and 59 per cent of the first-generation women were born of parents who were still Italian citizens at the time of the inquiry. Only about 5 per cent of the men and women among the second- and third-generation Italian Americans were born of Italian citizens.

Both parents were reported to be alive at the time of the inquiry by 44 per cent of the Italian subjects, 21 per cent of the first-generation Italian Americans and 62 per cent of the second- and third-generation Italian Americans. One parent was reported to be alive by 35 per cent, 21 per cent and 25 per cent of the three groups, respectively. Both parents were reported to be dead by 21 per cent, 57 per cent and 13 per cent, respectively.

The fathers of 46 per cent of the Italian subjects, 58 per cent of the first-generation Italian Americans, and 29 per cent of the second- and third-generation Italian Americans were known to be dead at the time of the interviews. In all groups, cardiovascular diseases ranked as the major cause of death, followed by digestive and respiratory diseases. War deaths were reported for 6 per cent of the Italian and less than 1 per cent of the Italian-American fathers, while accidental deaths were listed for 1 per cent of the Italian and 4 per cent of the Italian-American fathers.

The mothers of 28 per cent of the Italian subjects, 72 per cent

TABLE 3.—*Citizenship of Parents of Italian-American Subjects (in Per Cent)*

		ITALIAN AMERICANS				
		Male		*Female*		*Total*
FATHER	MOTHER	1st (*N=28*)	2d+3d (*N=81*)	1st (*N=44*)	2d+3d (*N=98*)	(*N=251*)
U.S.	U.S.	18	79	32	83	66
Italy	Italy	75	5	59	5	22
U.S.	Italy	4	2	0	1	2
Italy	U.S.	0	2	2	5	3
U.S.	No inf.	4	1	0	0	1
No inf.	U.S.	0	2	0	1	1
No inf.	No inf.	0	8	7	5	6
Totals		*101*	*99*	*100*	*100*	*101*

of the first-generation Italian Americans and 13 per cent of the second- and third-generation Italian Americans were known to be dead. The major cause of death was cardiovascular diseases, followed by cancer and respiratory diseases.

In all three groups, the mothers of the subjects were able to fill their roles for a longer period than were the fathers in shaping the personality of the subjects. At the time of death of their fathers, 20 per cent of the Italian subjects, 12 per cent of the first-generation Italian Americans and 13 per cent of the second- and third-generation Italian Americans were less than 20 years old. In contrast, only 10 per cent of the Italians, 8 per cent of the first-generation Italian Americans and 7 per cent of the second- and third-generation Italian Americans lost their mothers before the subjects reached the age of 20.

The marital status of the parents of the subjects is indicated in Table 4. Approximately the same proportion—42 per cent of the Italian parents and 48 per cent of the Italian-American parents—were described as alive and living together, and only 2 per cent of the Italian parents and 2 per cent of the Italian-American parents were married but separated. There were no cases of divorce in the Italian group, and only two among the Italian Americans.

These statistics do not necessarily indicate that marriage in the Italian culture is a more successful venture than in other cultures. They point to the fact, however, that divorce—even when legally possible—is seldom accepted as a solution to marital difficulties. Accordingly, within the framework of the Italian culture, the nutritional behavior of the child or adolescent will rarely be affected by any anxiety stemming from possible divorce of the parents.

Heights and Weights

The Italian-American subjects, in comparison with those in the Italian group, were appreciably taller and demonstrated a significantly greater tendency toward obesity.

Among the women, 43 per cent of the Italians but only 9 per cent of the first-generation and 6 per cent of the second- and third-generation Italian Americans were less than 5 feet in height. Among the men, 75 per cent of the Italians were less than 5 feet 6 inches in height, in contrast to 46 per cent of the first-generation and 14 per cent of the second- and third-generation Italian Americans. Similarly, only 2 per cent of the Italians but 4 per cent of the first-

TABLE 4.—*Marital Status of Parents of Subjects (in Per Cent)*

ITALIANS				ITALIAN AMERICANS				
Male	*Female*	*Total*		*Male*		*Female*		*Total*
				1st	2d+3d	1st	2d+3d	
(*N*=*125*)	(*N*=*122*)	(*N*=*247*)		(*N*=*28*)	(*N*=*81*)	(*N*=*44*)	(*N*=*98*)	(*N*=*251*)
35	50	42	Living together	14	64	25	53	48
2	1	2	Living apart	0	2	0	5	2
0	0	0	Divorced	0	1	0	0	1
6	7	7	Father widowed	4	5	14	5	6
1	0	1	Father widowed, remarried	4	2	5	0	2
22	24	23	Mother widowed	11	15	5	15	13
3	1	2	Mother widowed, remarried	0	1	0	5	2
28	14	20	Both dead	64	9	52	16	26
4	3	4	Incomplete information	4	0	0	0	0
101	*100*	*100*	*Totals*	*101*	*99*	*101*	*99*	*100*

TABLE 5.—*Weight Deviations of Subjects from "Ideal" (in Per Cent)*

Italians				Italian Americans				
Male	*Female*	*Total*		*Male*		*Female*		*Total*
				1st	2d+3d	1st	2d+3d	
(*N*=*125*)	(*N*=*122*)	(*N*=*247*)		(*N*=*28*)	(*N*=*81*)	(*N*=*44*)	(*N*=*98*)	(*N*=*251*)
11	8	10	Underweight 11.1–30%	0	4	2	7	4
18	20	18	Underweight 1–11%	4	14	9	27	17
13	2	8	"Ideal" weight	7	1	2	2	2
30	15	22	Overweight 1–10%	29	25	16	30	26
18	24	21	Overweight 10.1–20%	32	33	27	14	25
7	16	11	Overweight 20.1–30%	21	16	16	9	14
2	9	6	Overweight 30.1–40%	0	5	2	2	3
2	6	4	Overweight 40% or more	7	1	18	8	7
0	0	0	No information	0	1	7	1	2
101	*100*	*100*	*Totals*	*100*	*100*	*99*	*100*	*100*

generation and 21 per cent of the second- and third-generation Italian Americans were at least 6 feet tall.

In analyzing the weights of the subjects, the mean value of the weight range for medium-frame individuals as given in the Metropolitan Life Insurance Company tables was selected as the "ideal" weight for each height. Although this selection is arbitrary, it nevertheless permits a comparison of the relative frequency of underweight and overweight in the three groups.

On this basis, as shown in Table 5, some degree of underweight was found in 28 per cent of the Italians, 8 per cent of the first-generation Italian Americans, and 26 per cent of the second- and third-generation Italian Americans. The percentages of underweight men and women in the Italian group were essentially the same, but the incidence of underweight in both Italian-American groups was about twice as frequent among the women.

A significant degree of underweight, marked by deviations of 11 to 25 per cent below the "ideal," was noted in 10 per cent of the Italians and in 1 per cent of the first-generation and 6 per cent of the second- and third-generation Italian Americans.

Some degree of overweight was observed in 64 per cent of the Italians, 83 per cent of the first-generation Italian Americans, and 71 per cent of the second- and third-generation Italian Americans. This tendency toward obesity was considered to be significant, marked by deviations of 10 to 30 per cent above the "ideal," in 32 per cent of the Italians, 47 per cent of the first-generation Italian Americans, and 35 per cent of the second- and third-generation Italian Americans. An even more serious degree of overweight, marked by deviations of more than 30 per cent above the "ideal," was noted in 9 per cent of the Italians, 15 per cent of the first-generation Italian Americans, and 8 per cent of the second- and third-generation Italian Americans.

In the Italian group, significant obesity—indicated by deviations of more than 10 per cent above "ideal" weight—was found in 29 per cent of the men and 55 per cent of the women. Of the first-generation Italian Americans, 61 per cent of the men and 64 per cent of the women were involved. In the second- and third-generation group, 56 per cent of the men and 34 per cent of the women were involved.

Thus, the rate of marked obesity in Italian-American men appears to be about twice as high as in Italian men, and substantially

TABLE 6.—*Marital Status of Subjects (in Per Cent)*

	ITALIANS			ITALIAN AMERICANS				
	Male	*Female*	*Total*	*Male*		*Female*		*Total*
				1st	2d+3d	1st	2d+3d	
	(*N*=125)	(*N*=122)	(*N*=247)	(*N*=28)	(*N*=81)	(*N*=44)	(*N*=98)	(*N*=251)
Single	50	52	51	14	38	2	27	25
Married, living with spouse	47	37	42	75	62	75	61	65
Married, living apart	1	1	1	0	0	5	2	2
Legally separated	0	1	0	0	0	0	0	0
Divorced, not remarried	0	0	0	0	0	5	2	2
Divorced, remarried	0	0	0	4	0	2	3	2
Widowed, not remarried	1	8	4	4	0	11	5	4
Widowed, remarried	1	1	1	4	0	0	0	0
Totals	*100*	*100*	*99*	*101*	*100*	*100*	*100*	*100*

higher than in Italian-American women. The greater hazards accompanying obesity in males renders this situation particularly noteworthy.

Marital Status

The marital status of the subjects is indicated in Table 6.

The number of single men and women in the Italian group is disproportionate. The unavailability of married subjects in Italy for this study is chiefly responsible for the fact that the inquiry in that country was made largely on unmarried men and women.

It will be noted that none of the Italian subjects but nearly 4 per cent of the Italian Americans were divorced.

Of the 120 Italian subjects who had been married, 82 per cent reported having at least one child, while this was reported for 85 per cent of the 67 first-generation and 79 per cent of the 122 second- and third-generation Italian Americans who had been married.

Larger families, with three or more children, were reported by 19 per cent of the married Italian subjects, 46 per cent of the married first-generation Italian Americans, and 12 per cent of the married second- and third-generation Italian Americans. Differential age distribution accounts for much of this difference.

Religion

As noted earlier, the nutritional habits of an individual are believed to be based to a certain extent on attitudes and related emotions experienced by the individual beginning early in his psychological life. Among these phenomena, religious experiences may well be of high importance. Ritual fasting, for example, is usually a vital practice in many religions. The use or avoidance of certain foods is embodied in the laws of practically all religions. The ingestion of food is often linked with religious symbolism. Accordingly, it was felt essential to survey the religious attitudes and current religious practices of the subjects.

The overwhelming majority of these men and women were Catholics. Of the Italian subjects, more than 99 per cent were Catholics and all the married subjects were wedded to Catholics. Of the first-generation Italian Americans, 97 per cent were Catholics and the spouse of every married subject in the group was likewise a Catholic. Among the second- and third-generation Italian Americans, 94 per cent of the men and 90 per cent of the women were Catholics. One per cent of the Catholic men and 5 per cent of the Catholic women had married a spouse of a different faith.

Information on any but the most superficial aspects of religious participation is rather difficult to obtain in any circle, especially in such a group as the Italian subjects studied here, who consider experiences connected with religious participation to be quite intimate. The average Italian and, to a certain extent, the average Italian American observed in this investigation were reluctant to disclose what they considered an experience totally unrelated to health and perhaps unrelated even to emotional problems in general.

The data obtained in this area are presented in Table 7. They do not give a complete picture of the religious attitudes and practices of the subjects, for they indicate primarily participation in such solemn functions as the Mass and other rituals. Nevertheless, they may serve as a basis of comparison between the groups.

No participation in religious activities was reported by 8 per cent of the Italian subjects, 10 per cent of the first-generation Italian Americans and 4 per cent of the second- and third-generation Italian Americans. This lack of participation was reported more frequently by Italian men than women. Among the Italian Americans, however, it was reported by 7 per cent of the men and 11 per cent of the women in the first generation, and 2 per cent of the men and 5 per cent of the women in the second- and third-generation group.

It must be kept in mind that the Italians who declared that they never go to church would, in the same breath, state that they were Catholics. None of them would refuse participation in such fundamental rituals of Catholicism as baptism, confirmation, marriage and burial in consecrated ground.

These statistics, pointing to a striking increase in religious activity by both men and women from the first generation of Italian Americans to the second and third, appear to be extremely significant. Whether this trend is related to a reawakening of religious feelings or more to an understanding of the social implications of religious attendance remains to be seen.

Once-a-week church attendance was commonly reported more frequently by women than by men—54 per cent of the men and 84 per cent of the women among the Italians, 29 per cent of the

TABLE 7.–*Frequency of Church Attendance by Subjects and Spouses (in Per Cent)*

Italians: *Male*	Italians: *Female*	Italians: *Total*		Italian Americans: *Male* 1st	Italian Americans: *Male* 2d+3d	Italian Americans: *Female* 1st	Italian Americans: *Female* 2d+3d	Italian Americans: *Total*
(*N*=125)	(*N*=122)	(*N*=247)	SUBJECTS	(*N*=28)	(*N*=81)	(*N*=44)	(*N*=98)	(*N*=251)
14	1	8	Never	7	2	11	5	6
13	3	8	1–4 times a year	43	21	9	10	17
4	2	3	5–10 times a year	4	10	5	5	6
10	5	7	1–2 times a month	14	16	9	5	10
54	84	68	About once a week	29	38	39	51	42
1	5	3	More than once a week	4	9	25	20	15
5	0	2	No information	0	4	2	3	3
101	*100*	99	*Totals*	*101*	*100*	*100*	99	99
(*N*=62)	(*N*=58)	(*N*=120)	SPOUSES	(*N*=23)	(*N*=50)	(*N*=36)	(*N*=65)	(*N*=174)
4	3	4	Never	9	0	17	18	11
4	3	4	1–4 times a year	4	18	30	26	21
4	5	4	5–10 times a year	0	12	5	12	9
4	13	8	1–2 times a month	22	14	5	6	10
73	67	70	About once a week	61	44	25	25	35
2	2	2	More than once a week	0	6	14	6	7
8	8	8	No information	4	6	5	6	6
99	*101*	*100*	*Totals*	*100*	*100*	99	99	99

men and 39 per cent of the women among the first-generation Italian Americans, and 38 per cent of the men and 51 per cent of the women among the second- and third-generation group. The increasing frequency of this pattern from the first generation in this country to the second and third is noteworthy.

More active participation, as evidenced by church attendance more than once a week, was observed in only 3 per cent of the Italians but 15 per cent of the Italian Americans. In all groups, this pattern was found more commonly among the women than the men.

One of the most valuable findings concerns the change in religious attitudes as expressed by men and women. In Italy, it would appear that there is a rather large percentage of men whose religious participation is, so to say, by proxy. This does not imply male hostility against the religion in which they were born, or any denial of it. Among Italians, there appears to be little of the heated attitude for or against religion which is often observed in other groups, both Catholic and non-Catholic. Nevertheless, within the framework of the Italian culture, religious participation appears to be a need felt significantly more deeply by the women, and it is the women who are by far the most active participants in religious activities. In the Italian-American groups, however, there is a clear trend toward disappearance of these differences between men and women.

This trend is further supported by data on the religious participation of the spouses of the married subjects, also presented in Table 7. Among the first-generation Italian Americans, once-a-week church attendance was reported by 25 per cent of the husbands of female subjects and 61 per cent of the wives of male subjects. In the second- and third-generation group, such participation was noted by 25 per cent of the husbands of female subjects and 44 per cent of the wives of male subjects.

Further differences became apparent when the subjects compared their own religious participation with that of their parents. The great majority of Italian subjects declared that their religious activity was more or less the same as that of their parents. No such pattern was found among the Italian Americans, with one sizable group reporting less religious activity than their parents, another reporting about the same activity, and a third reporting more. These findings in the Italian-American subjects can hardly be considered indicative of changes in religious feelings; they hint more of adaptations to the social standards of different communities.

Language

The language spoken and understood by all subjects in Italy was, as expected, Italian.

Among the first-generation Italian Americans, 93 per cent of the men and 91 per cent of the women spoke and understood both Italian and English, while 3 per cent of the men and 5 per cent of the women spoke and understood only Italian.

Among the second- and third-generation Italian Americans, 64 per cent of the men and 66 per cent of the women spoke and understood both languages, while 22 per cent of the men and 17 per cent of the women spoke and understood only English. In addition, 14 per cent of both the men and the women in this group spoke only English but could understand Italian.

Education

The number of years of formal education completed by the subjects is given in Table 8.

In the Italian group, 82 per cent of the subjects completed 8 years of schooling, 28 per cent completed 12 years, and 20 per cent completed 16 years. It must be emphasized that these data do not serve as an index to Italian education. The subjects in Italy were selected in such a way that their educational status more closely approached that of the Italian Americans.

In the first-generation Italian-American group, grammar school was completed by 42 per cent, high school by 18 per cent, and college by 4 per cent. The corresponding values for the second- and third-generation subjects are 90, 61 and 11 per cent, respectively.

In all groups, those subjects who did not complete a stage of education gave financial reasons as the major cause for leaving school.

Economic Status

The occupations of the male subjects, and of husbands of female subjects, are shown in Table 9. It can be seen that 51 per cent of the Italian men, 22 per cent of the first-generation Italian Americans and 34 per cent of the second- and third-generation Italian Americans can be classified as white-collar workers; 10 per cent of the Italians, 61 per cent of the first-generation and 52 per cent of the

TABLE 8.—*Education of Subjects (in Per Cent)*

Italians *Male*	Italians *Female*	Italians *Total*		Italian Americans *Male* 1st	Italian Americans *Male* 2d+3d	Italian Americans *Female* 1st	Italian Americans *Female* 2d+3d	Italian Americans *Total*
(*N*=*125*)	(*N*=*122*)	(*N*=*247*)		(*N*=28)	(*N*=*81*)	(*N*=*44*)	(*N*=98)	(*N*=*251*)
1	0	1	None	4	0	5	0	1
6	6	6	1–4 years	35	1	32	1	10
14	4	10	5–7 years	18	6	18	10	11
29	65	46	8 years	11	10	11	9	10
10	7	8	9–11 years	18	25	9	14	18
3	2	2	12 years	4	25	14	44	28
10	2	6	13–15 years	7	15	2	15	12
8	0	4	16 years	0	9	2	2	4
6	7	6	Prof. or grad. study	4	7	0	0	3
10	8	10	Prof. or grad. degree	0	1	2	4	2
3	0	2	No information	0	1	5	0	1
100	*101*	*101*	*Totals*	*101*	*100*	*100*	*99*	*100*

TABLE 9.—*Occupations of Male Subjects and Husbands of Female Subjects (in Per Cent)*

Italians: *Male Subjects*	Italians: *Husbands*	Italians: *Total*		Italian Americans: *Male Subjects* 1st	Italian Americans: *Male Subjects* 2d+3d	Italian Americans: *Husbands* 1st	Italian Americans: *Husbands* 2d+3d	Italian Americans: *Total*
(*N*=*125*)	(*N*=*48*)	(*N*=*173*)		(*N*=*28*)	(*N*=*81*)	(*N*=*36*)	(*N*=*65*)	(*N*=*210*)
2	5	3	Professional, executive	14	9	13	18	14
38	52	42	Clerk	0	19	8	15	13
3	4	3	Salesman	4	0	3	9	4
2	5	3	Civil service	4	6	6	5	5
10	11	10	Skilled, semiskilled	61	52	53	45	51
20	22	20	Unskilled	8	0	8	2	3
16	0	12	Student	0	12	0	0	5
7	0	5	Unemployed	8	2	3	5	4
1	0	1	No information	0	0	6	2	1
99	*99*	*99*	*Totals*	*99*	*100*	*100*	*101*	*100*

second- and third-generation Italian Americans as skilled or semi-skilled workers; and 20 per cent of the Italians, 8 per cent of the first-generation and less than 1 per cent of the second- and third-generation Italian Americans as unskilled workers. The occupations of the husbands of female subjects are substantially the same in the several categories, the differences in the white-collar category being accounted for by the inclusion of students among the Italian and the second- and third-generation Italian-American subjects.

The occupations of the female subjects, and of wives of male subjects, are given in Table 10. It may be noted that 61 per cent of the Italians, 65 per cent of the first-generation Italian Americans and 86 per cent of the second- and third-generation Italian Americans were housewives; 28 per cent of the Italians, 10 per cent of the first-generation and 35 per cent of the second- and third-generation Italian Americans were white-collar workers; and less than 1 per cent of the Italians but 14 per cent of the first-generation and 6 per cent of the second- and third-generation Italian Americans were factory workers. Among the wives of first-generation Italian-American subjects 22 per cent were factory workers, compared to only 4 per cent in the second and third generations.

Nearly 85 per cent of the Italian subjects lived in a rented house or apartment, in contrast to 39 per cent of the first-generation and 41 per cent of the second- and third-generation Italian Americans. Only 10 per cent of the Italians lived in their own home, as contrasted to 43 per cent of the first-generation and 25 per cent of the second- and third-generation Italian Americans. None of the Italians but 8 per cent of the first-generation and 32 per cent of the second- and third-generation Italian Americans—a relatively younger group—lived with relatives.

Although 40 per cent of the Italian subjects possessed a telephone, only 1 per cent owned an automobile. In striking contrast, 85 per cent of the first-generation Italian Americans and 89 per cent of the second- and third-generation subjects possessed a telephone; 56 per cent of the first- and 76 per cent of the second- and third-generation subjects owned an automobile; 61 per cent of the first- and 71 per cent of the second- and third-generation subjects had a television set; and 40 per cent of the first- and 57 per cent of the second- and third-generation Italian Americans had all three.

Although 39 per cent of the Italians were carrying some form of insurance, none was paying for any purchases on the installment

TABLE 10.—*Occupations of Female Subjects and Wives of Male Subjects (in Per Cent)*

Italians: *Wives*	Italians: *Female Subjects*	Italians: *Total*		Italian Americans: *Wives*		Italian Americans: *Female Subjects*		Italian Americans: *Total*
				1st	2d+3d	1st	2d+3d	
(*N*=*61*)	(*N*=*122*)	(*N*=*183*)		(*N*=*23*)	(*N*=*50*)	(*N*=*44*)	(*N*=*98*)	(*N*=*215*)
74	54	61	Housewife	65	86	57	52	62
0	13	9	Professional, executive	0	2	5	12	7
20	14	16	Secretary, clerk	9	4	5	21	13
1	1	1	Saleswoman	4	4	0	2	2
0	1	1	Factory worker	22	4	14	6	9
0	2	1	Domestic	0	0	0	1	0
1	9	7	Other	0	0	9	2	3
0	7	4	None or unemployed	0	0	11	2	3
3	0	1	No information	0	0	0	1	0
99	*101*	*101*	*Totals*	*100*	*100*	*101*	*99*	*99*

plan. Among the first-generation Italian Americans, 47 per cent were carrying insurance, 7 per cent were buying on the installment plan, and 19 per cent were doing both. Among the second- and third-generation subjects, 39 per cent were carrying insurance, 2 per cent were buying on the installment plan, and 39 per cent were doing both.

Medical Status[1]

No subjects with major illnesses were accepted for this study, either in Italy or the United States. Minor physiological ailments, however, were detected in 16 (13 per cent) of the Italian men; in 16 (13 per cent) of the Italian women; in 34 (31 per cent) of the Italian-American men; and in 46 (32 per cent) of the Italian-American women.

The higher incidence of these minor illnesses in the Italian-American group cannot be construed as evidence that the health of Italians is generally better than that of Italian Americans. Instead, the difference here is due chiefly to the greater difficulty in obtaining Italian-American subjects for this investigation, and consequent acceptance of more subjects who were not physiologically perfect. In part it may be related also to the age difference between the groups: 47 per cent of the Italians were under 30 and only 9 per cent 50 years or over, whereas among the Italian Americans the corresponding percentages were 33 and 18.

In the Italian group, the subjects with minor disorders were classified as follows: cardiovascular, 3 men and 4 women; digestive, 10 men and 8 women; respiratory, 1 woman; metabolic, 1 man and 2 women; endocrine, 1 man; nutritional deficiency, 1 man; and reproductive, 1 woman.

In the Italian-American group, the classes were as follows: cardiovascular, 17 men and 25 women; digestive, 6 men and 7 women; respiratory, 3 men and 2 women; metabolic, 2 men and 2 women; endocrine, 4 men and 6 women; nutritional deficiency, 1 man; reproductive, 3 women; and allergic, 1 man and 1 woman.

A preliminary psychiatric survey indicated that 16 (13 per cent) of the Italian men and 5 (4 per cent) of the Italian women were facing nonpsychotic emotional difficulties. A similar impression was

[1] The incidence of diabetes and pre-diabetes in the subjects is not included here but will be discussed in a separate section in Chapter 5.

obtained in 13 (12 per cent) of the men and 29 (20 per cent) of the women in the Italian-American group.

The fact that 87 per cent of the Italian subjects exhibited no sign of physiological deviation and 90 per cent showed no serious emotional problems is particularly important. Its significance will become ever more apparent when it is noted that the overwhelming proportion of these subjects were regular users of wine. It is evident that the use of this alcoholic beverage, sometimes in considerable amounts, did not affect their health unfavorably.

Chapter 3

EATING HABITS

EARLY in this inquiry it became apparent that most of the subjects knew about their earliest eating patterns and could speak readily about them. Thus, the overwhelming majority of the subjects—96 per cent of the Italians and 92 per cent of the Italian Americans—reported at once that they had been breast fed during infancy. Interestingly, only about 1 per cent of the subjects in each group were unable to supply information on this experience of the distant past—an indication that such an early nutritional fact, closely linking mother and child psychologically, was discussed openly in the families of most Italians and Italian Americans.

More information was obtained on the present habits and attitudes of the subjects. Data on eating patterns, caloric intake and consumption of the basic food substances are given in the following sections.

Patterns of Eating

In their present eating patterns, 85 per cent of the Italians can be considered as "regular eaters," taking three meals a day at almost the same time daily with little or no change in the pattern of regular meals. Only 71 per cent of the first-generation and 47 per cent of the second- and third-generation Italian Americans can be so classified.

In the Italian group, a "regular" eating pattern was found in essentially the same proportion of men and women, presumably because of the widespread habit of sharing all three meals, including luncheon, with the family.[1]

Among the Italian Americans, this "regular" pattern was noted in 82 per cent of the men and 64 per cent of the women in the first generation, and in 47 per cent of the men and 47 per cent of the women in the second- and third-generation groups. In the subjects studied here, the increasing occurrence of a sporadic eating habit is related largely to the lack of a set time for luncheon.

The custom of consuming the largest meals on Sunday was obvious for the Italian Americans, but not for the Italians, who gen-

[1] Cf. Part II.

TABLE 11.—*Average Daily Caloric Intake (in Per Cent)*

Italians Male	Italians Female	Italians Total		Italian Americans Male 1st	Italian Americans Male 2d+3d	Italian Americans Female 1st	Italian Americans Female 2d+3d	Italian Americans Total
(N=125)	(N=122)	(N=247)		(N=28)	(N=81)	(N=44)	(N=98)	(N=251)
2	21	11	1,000–1,999	4	6	39	26	19
51	71	61	2,000–2,999	61	25	52	62	48
35	7	21	3,000–3,999	36	48	7	12	26
10	1	5	4,000–4,999	0	20	0	0	6
2	0	1	5,000 or more	0	1	0	0	0
0	0	0	No information	0	0	2	0	0
100	*100*	*99*	*Totals*	*101*	*99*	*100*	*100*	*99*

TABLE 12.—*Maximum 1-Day Caloric Intake (in Per Cent)*

Italians Male	Italians Female	Italians Total		Italian Americans Male 1st	Italian Americans Male 2d+3d	Italian Americans Female 1st	Italian Americans Female 2d+3d	Italian Americans Total
(N=125)	(N=122)	(N=247)		(N=28)	(N=81)	(N=44)	(N=98)	(N=251)
0	2	1	1,500–1,999	0	2	11	7	6
3	25	14	2,000–2,499	0	1	23	16	10
11	30	20	2,500–2,999	21	5	23	22	17
31	24	27	3,000–3,499	7	9	18	20	15
24	15	19	3,500–3,999	43	21	14	24	23
11	4	8	4,000–4,499	21	20	7	3	11
9	1	6	4,500–4,999	4	14	2	6	7
5	0	2	5,000–5,499	0	15	0	0	5
5	0	2	5,500 or more	4	14	0	1	5
1	0	0	No information	0	0	2	0	0
100	*101*	*99*	*Totals*	*100*	*101*	*100*	*99*	*99*

erally spaced their daily caloric intake more evenly through the week. Friday, generally considered to be the day on which small meals are consumed by Catholics, was named as the day on which 19 per cent of the Italians and 23 per cent of the Italian Americans ingested the lowest number of calories.

Caloric Intake

The average daily caloric intake of the subjects is shown in Table 11.

A further analysis indicated that 84 (33 per cent) of the Italians had an average daily intake of 2,300 calories or more and thus could be classified as "heavy" eaters, as could 39 (54 per cent) of the first-generation and 121 (67 per cent) of the second- and third-generation Italian Americans.

The largest number of calories consumed on any one day during the week of observation is indicated in Table 12. Only 1 per cent of the Italian subjects—2 women—never exceeded 2,000 calories daily, in comparison to 6 per cent of the Italian Americans—2 men and 12 women. In contrast, 4 per cent of the Italians—all men—ate more than 5,000 calories on one day, as did 10 per cent of the Italian Americans—24 men and 1 women.

The smallest number of calories consumed on any one day is shown in Table 13. It can be seen that 8 per cent of the Italians and 27 per cent of the Italian Americans ate less than 1,400 calories on at least one day of the week. About three-quarters of these "light" eaters in both groups were women.

These findings confirm an impression which is apparently valid for groups and nationalities practically all over the world. For a variety of reasons, provided weight, height and physiological needs are equal, women eat less than men. In the group of subjects observed here, two factors seem to prevail: first, women may limit their diet for aesthetic reasons; and second, the men who do heavy manual work need more calories than do the women who stay at home. In addition, as will be noted later, the significant caloric contribution of alcohol to the diet of male Italians may play an important role.

Proteins, Fats, Carbohydrates

Analysis of the meals eaten by the subjects demonstrated that the men in all groups had a higher average daily intake of protein

TABLE 13.—*Minimum 1-Day Caloric Intake (in Per Cent)*

Italians				Italian Americans				
Male	*Female*	*Total*		*Male*		*Female*		*Total*
				1st	2d+3d	1st	2d+3d	
(*N*=*125*)	(*N*=*122*)	(*N*=*247*)		(*N*=*28*)	(*N*=*81*)	(*N*=*44*)	(*N*=*98*)	(*N*=*251*)
1	0	1	Less than 350	0	1	5	1	1
0	0	0	350–699	0	0	2	3	1
1	1	1	700–1,049	11	5	14	9	9
3	8	6	1,050–1,399	7	9	18	23	16
5	28	16	1,400–1,749	21	10	32	22	20
18	37	27	1,750–2,099	14	20	16	24	20
30	18	23	2,100–2,449	29	17	5	8	13
20	5	13	2,450–2,799	14	10	7	5	8
9	2	5	2,800–3,149	4	10	0	4	5
5	1	3	3,150–3,499	0	10	0	0	3
8	1	5	3,500 or more	0	9	0	0	3
1	0	0	No information	0	0	2	0	0
101	*101*	*100*	*Totals*	*100*	*101*	*101*	*99*	*99*

TABLE 14.—*Average Daily Protein Intake in Grams (in Per Cent)*

Italians				Italian Americans				
Male	*Female*	*Total*		*Male*		*Female*		*Total*
				1st	2d+3d	1st	2d+3d	
(*N*=125)	(*N*=122)	(*N*=247)		(*N*=28)	(*N*=81)	(*N*=44)	(*N*=98)	(*N*=251)
0	0	0	20–39	0	1	2	0	1
1	6	3	40–59	0	1	9	5	4
9	35	22	60–79	7	1	36	30	19
27	45	36	80–99	25	12	25	37	25
31	10	21	100–119	32	26	18	16	22
20	3	12	120–139	21	26	7	10	16
9	1	5	140–159	11	19	0	2	8
3	0	2	160 or more	4	14	0	0	5
0	0	0	No information	0	0	2	0	0
100	*100*	*101*	*Totals*	*100*	*100*	*99*	*100*	*100*

TABLE 15.—*Average Daily Fat Intake in Grams (in Per Cent)*

Italians				Italian Americans				
Male	*Female*	*Total*		*Male*		*Female*		*Total*
				1st	2d+3d	1st	2d+3d	
(*N*=125)	(*N*=122)	(*N*=247)		(*N*=28)	(*N*=81)	(*N*=44)	(*N*=98)	(*N*=251)
2	2	2	Less than 50	4	1	9	1	3
68	76	71	50–99	43	12	61	47	38
27	21	24	100–149	50	47	20	42	41
3	1	2	150–199	4	32	5	9	15
0	0	0	200 or more	0	7	2	1	3
0	0	0	No information	0	0	2	0	0
100	*100*	*99*	*Totals*	*101*	*99*	*99*	*100*	*100*

than did the women, as shown in Table 14, and that the ingestion of protein foods was substantially higher among the Italian Americans than among the Italians. Thus, 40 per cent of the Italians, 42 per cent of the first-generation and 54 per cent of the second- and third-generation Italian Americans consumed more than 100 g. of protein daily.

Similarly, as shown in Table 15, men consumed more fat than women, and Italian Americans more than Italians. It may be noted that 26 per cent of the Italians, 37 per cent of the first-generation and 68 per cent of the second- and third-generation Italian Americans ate more than 100 g. of fat daily.

The intake of carbohydrates, as shown in Table 16, was likewise higher among men than among women, but these foods were used in larger quantities by the Italians than by the Italian Americans. A daily consumption of more than 400 g. was reported by 22 per cent of the Italians, 8 per cent of the first-generation and 16 per cent of the second- and third-generation Italian Americans.

A more detailed examination demonstrated that the carbohydrates obtained by the Italian subjects were from the more slowly absorbable carbohydrate foods such as breadstuffs, cereals and rice, while the Italian Americans were more likely to indulge in the highly soluble and more quickly absorbable sugars.

The prevalence of slowly absorbable carbohydrates in the diets of the Italian subjects seems to supply some measure of stability to blood sugar levels. On the other hand, the ingestion of rapidly absorbable carbohydrates would permit wide and frequent fluctuations of blood sugar concentrations and therefore allow major or minor hypoglycemic crises. In this connection it may be worth while to recall that a relationship seems to exist between elevated blood sugar concentrations and resistance of the central nervous system to the most toxic effects of such substances as alcohol (3). Accordingly, in comparison with the Italian Americans, the dietary habits of the Italians appear to afford a greater protection against reactions resulting from the ingestion of large amounts of alcoholic beverages.

Geographical Origin and Intake of Foodstuffs

An analysis of the mean total daily caloric intake of the subjects according to their origins in Northern, Central and Southern Italy disclosed a generally lower value for those of Southern extraction.

TABLE 16.—*Average Daily Carbohydrate Intake in Grams (in Per Cent)*

	ITALIANS			ITALIAN AMERICANS				
	Male	*Female*	*Total*	*Male*		*Female*		*Total*
				1st	2d+3d	1st	2d+3d	
	(*N*=125)	(*N*=122)	(*N*=247)	(*N*=28)	(*N*=81)	(*N*=44)	(*N*=98)	(*N*=251)
Less than 200	0	7	3	14	4	32	22	17
200–299	20	50	34	32	25	48	52	40
300–399	44	37	40	43	41	11	21	28
400–499	22	4	13	11	27	7	3	12
500–599	6	2	4	0	2	0	1	2
600–699	5	1	3	0	1	0	0	0
700 or more	4	0	2	0	0	0	0	0
No information	0	0	0	0	0	2	0	0
Totals	*101*	*101*	99	*100*	*100*	*100*	99	99

Among the Italians, the caloric intake[2] in the three areas, respectively, was 3,180±107, 3,080±97, and 2,960±122 for the men, and 2,410±76, 2,460±101, and 2,380±61 for the women.

Among the Northern, Central and Southern subjects of the first-generation Italian-American group, the corresponding values were 2,980±163, 3,060±143, and 2,550±127 for the men, and 2,330±107, 2,040±110, and 1,640±248 for the women.

In the second- and third-generation group, the values were 3,560 ±131, 3,430±252, and 3,090±126 for the men, and 2,320±90, 2,270 ±86, and 2,320±96 for the women.

So far as protein intake is concerned, no significant regional differences were observed among the Italians, daily values of 107 to 112 g. being calculated for the men and 82 to 86 g. for the women. In the Italian-American group, however, subjects of Southern extraction reported relatively lower values.

Among the first-generation subjects, the daily protein intake in grams calculated for those of Northern, Central and Southern origin was 123±9.0, 123±10.2, and 105±5.9 for the men, and 93±4.6, 82 ±4.0 and 66±7.8 for the women.

Among the second- and third-generation subjects, the values were 135±5.3, 131±9.5 and 120±4.8 for the men, and 90±2.8, 91±4.4 and 89±3.8 for the women.

No significant relation was found between geographic origin and fat intake by the Italians, but a marked increase in fat consumption was noted from the first- to the second- and third-generation Italian Americans of Central and Southern extraction.

For the Italians, the daily intake of fats in grams was calculated to be 96±3.6, 85±3.6, and 90±3.8 for the men of Northern, Central and Southern origin, respectively, and 85±3.4, 82±3.5, and 86±2.7 for the women.

Among the first-generation Italian Americans, the values were 103±4.5, 88±11.0, and 111±9.5 for the men, and 104±7.9, 77±7.0, and 72±11.7 for the women.

Among the second- and third-generation subjects, the values were 154±5.8, 153±15.6, and 134±6.2 for the men, and 104±5.0, 99±5.3, and 107±6.6 for the women.

A detailed study of carbohydrate consumption indicated a generally lower intake by subjects of Southern extraction, and a relatively

[2] The values in the present section are given as means and standard errors of the means.

TABLE 17.—*Average Daily Calcium Intake in Milligrams (in Per Cent)*

Italians				Italian Americans				
Male	*Female*	*Total*		*Male*		*Female*		*Total*
				1st	2d+3d	1st	2d+3d	
(*N*=*125*)	(*N*=*122*)	(*N*=*247*)		(*N*=*28*)	(*N*=*81*)	(*N*=*44*)	(*N*=*98*)	(*N*=*251*)
9	13	11	Less than 400	4	2	7	6	5
26	36	31	400–599	14	7	16	15	13
30	27	28	600–799	25	22	32	37	30
20	15	18	800–999	25	22	30	14	21
14	7	10	1,000–1,199	21	16	9	18	16
1	2	1	1,200–1,399	4	16	2	3	7
0	0	0	1,400–1,599	7	4	2	1	3
0	1	0	1,600 or more	0	10	0	5	5
0	0	0	No information	0	0	2	0	0
100	*101*	99	*Totals*	*100*	99	*100*	99	*100*

TABLE 18.—*Average Daily Iron Intake in Milligrams (in Per Cent)*

Italians				Italian Americans				
Male	*Female*	*Total*		*Male*		*Female*		*Total*
				1st	2d+3d	1st	2d+3d	
(*N*=*125*)	(*N*=*122*)	(*N*=*247*)		(*N*=*28*)	(*N*=*81*)	(*N*=*44*)	(*N*=*98*)	(*N*=*251*)
0	0	0	1–4	0	1	0	0	0
17	36	26	5–9	0	4	11	11	7
42	50	46	10–14	21	14	48	51	35
24	10	17	15–19	39	37	30	31	34
10	2	6	20–24	32	26	5	6	15
8	2	5	25 or more	7	19	5	1	8
0	0	0	No information	0	0	2	0	0
101	*100*	*100*	*Totals*	99	*101*	*101*	*100*	99

lower intake by most first-generation Italian Americans as compared both to Italians and to second- and third-generation Italian Americans.

In the Italian group, the daily intake of carbohydrates in grams was calculated to be 412±21.2, 395±17.1, and 354±14.8 for the men of Northern, Central and Southern origin, respectively, and 301±10.2, 310±21.0, and 289±8.1 for the women.

Among the first-generation Italian Americans, the values were 313±31.0, 363±24.2, and 264±15.7 for the men, and 276±17.6, 230 ±13.0, and 179±26.9 for the women.

Among the second- and third-generation group, the values were 384±17.8, 367±32.2, and 337±14.5 for the men, and 260±12.0, 255 ±10.5, and 260±13.4 for the women.

Minerals and Vitamins

As shown in Table 17, a substantial proportion of the subjects in all groups fell below the recommended calcium intake of 1,000 mg. per day (24). This deficiency was most marked among the Italian subjects, affecting 85 per cent of the men and 91 per cent of the women. Among the Italian Americans, it was observed in 68 per cent of the men and 85 per cent of the women in the first-generation and in 53 per cent of the men and 72 per cent of the women in the second- and third-generation groups.

The intake of iron is shown in Table 18. It can be seen that 17 per cent of the men and 36 per cent of the women in the Italian group reported an average daily intake of less than 10 mg. In contrast, none of the men and only 11 per cent of the women of the first-generation Italian Americans, and 5 per cent of the men and 11 per cent of the women of the second- and third-generation group had such a low intake of iron.

The intake of Vitamin A by the Italian group was not determined. Among the Italian Americans, 18 per cent of the men and 27 per cent of the women in the first-generation group ingested less than the recommended 5,000 I.U. per day, as did 36 per cent of the men and 34 per cent of the women in the second- and third-generation group.

In the case of Vitamin B_1, as shown in Table 19, a substantial number of Italian subjects failed to meet minimum daily requirements. While 64 per cent of the Italians reported an average daily intake of less than 1 mg., this was noted in only 10 per cent of

TABLE 19.—*Average Daily Vitamin B_1 Intake in Milligrams (in Per Cent)*

Italians				Italian Americans				
Male	*Female*	*Total*		*Male*		*Female*		*Total*
				1st	2d+3d	1st	2d+3d	
(*N*=*125*)	(*N*=*122*)	(*N*=*247*)		(*N*=*28*)	(*N*=*81*)	(*N*=*44*)	(*N*=*98*)	(*N*=*251*)
48	82	64	Less than 1.0	4	2	14	12	8
42	15	29	1.0–1.9	32	26	66	61	47
7	3	5	2.0–2.9	61	46	16	26	34
2	0	2	3.0–3.9	4	26	2	1	10
0	0	0	No information	0	0	2	0	0
99	*100*	*100*	*Totals*	*101*	*100*	*100*	*100*	99

TABLE 20.—*Average Daily Riboflavin Intake in Milligrams (in Per Cent)*

Italians				Italian Americans				
Male	*Female*	*Total*		*Male*		*Female*		*Total*
				1st	2d+3d	1st	2d+3d	
(*N*=*125*)	(*N*=*122*)	(*N*=*247*)		(*N*=*28*)	(*N*=*81*)	(*N*=*44*)	(*N*=*98*)	(*N*=*251*)
10	24	17	Less than 1.0	0	2	5	2	2
66	62	64	1.0–1.9	39	10	52	51	37
10	6	8	2.0–2.9	43	56	25	38	42
1	1	1	3.0–3.9	7	25	9	8	14
3	3	3	4.0–4.9	11	5	7	1	4
10	4	7	5.0 or more	0	2	0	0	1
0	0	0	No information	0	0	2	0	0
100	*100*	*100*	*Totals*	*100*	*100*	*100*	*100*	*100*

TABLE 21.—*Average Daily Niacin Intake in Milligrams (in Per Cent)*

ITALIANS				ITALIAN AMERICANS				
Male	*Female*	*Total*		*Male*		*Female*		*Total*
				1st	2d+3d	1st	2d+3d	
(*N*=*125*)	(*N*=*122*)	(*N*=*247*)		(*N*=*28*)	(*N*=*81*)	(*N*=*44*)	(*N*=*98*)	(*N*=*251*)
10	31	21	5–9	0	2	2	0	1
39	53	46	10–14	4	0	23	27	14
25	10	18	15–19	21	11	39	41	29
15	3	10	20–24	18	27	23	22	24
10	2	6	25–29	57	59	11	10	31
0	0	0	No information	0	0	2	0	0
99	*99*	*101*	*Totals*	*100*	*99*	*100*	*100*	*99*

TABLE 22.—*Average Daily Vitamin C Intake in Milligrams (in Per Cent)*

ITALIANS				ITALIAN AMERICANS				
Male	*Female*	*Total*		*Male*		*Female*		*Total*
				1st	2d+3d	1st	2d+3d	
(*N*=*125*)	(*N*=*122*)	(*N*=*247*)		(*N*=*28*)	(*N*=*81*)	(*N*=*44*)	(*N*=*98*)	(*N*=*251*)
24	12	18	1–49	21	12	14	13	14
38	56	46	50–99	25	41	41	40	38
19	20	20	100–149	46	31	25	29	31
14	7	10	150–199	0	12	14	13	11
5	4	5	200 or more	7	4	5	5	5
0	0	0	No information	0	0	2	0	0
100	*99*	*99*	*Totals*	*99*	*100*	*101*	*100*	*99*

the first-generation and 8 per cent of the second- and third-generation Italian Americans.

A somewhat similar situation exists with respect to riboflavin, as indicated in Table 20, with 17 per cent of the Italians reporting an average daily intake of less than 1 mg., compared to 3 per cent of the first-generation and 2 per cent of the second- and third-generation Italian Americans.

The data on daily niacin intake, presented in Table 21, indicate that 49 per cent of the men and 84 per cent of the women in the Italian group ingested less than the recommended amount of this vitamin. This deficit was found in 4 per cent of the men and 25 per cent of the women in the first-generation and in 2 per cent of the men and 27 per cent of the women in the second- and third-generation Italian-American groups.

In the case of Vitamin C, as shown in Table 22, 24 per cent of the men and 12 per cent of the women among the Italians were definitely below recommended levels, as were 21 per cent of the men and 14 per cent of the women in the first-generation and 12 per cent of the men and 13 per cent of the women in the second- and third-generation Italian-American groups.

So far as most of the minerals and vitamins discussed here are concerned, apparent deficiencies are obviously more common among the women in each group. This may be attributed at least in part to the self-directed reducing diets being undertaken by more and more women. On the other hand, it should be noted that practically none of these subjects—male or female—demonstrated any signs of significant nutritional deficiency, and that the so-called deficiencies here may be more relative than actual.

Chapter 4

CONSUMPTION OF FLUIDS

WHEN an infant's nutritional patterns are first established, distinctions between solid and liquid food are, for all practical purposes, nonexistent. For the infant, milk is neither solid nor liquid. The dichotomy between what is solid and what is liquid results from the process of growth, and is deeply affected by psychological and social factors.

Thereafter, as the individual progresses toward adult life, there is not merely a distinction between solid and liquid but often a failure to recognize the importance of liquids. In past nutritional inquiries, for example, attention has seldom been paid to the total amount of fluids ingested by the subjects.

This topic, however, is of enormous significance. Fluids in general represent fundamental food items, required for the maintenance of the individual's internal environment and for his very survival.

Furthermore, where the problems of alcoholism are concerned, data on the ingestion of all fluids—including water, milk, coffee, fruit juices and soft drinks—have a special bearing. Since alcoholism may well be considered as an extreme deviation of a normal drinking habit, study of the use of these nonalcoholic fluids should not be neglected.

Total Fluids

The weekly ingestion of all fluids—alcoholic as well as nonalcoholic beverages—by all the subjects is indicated in Table 23.

The increasing use of such fluids by the Italian-American subjects is striking. Thus, 14 per cent of the Italians but none of the Italian Americans consumed less than 100 oz. during the week; 47 per cent of the Italians and 4 per cent of the Italian Americans consumed between 100 and 200 oz.; 31 per cent of the Italians and 24 per cent of the Italian Americans consumed between 200 and 300 oz.; 6 per cent of the Italians and 32 per cent of the Italian Americans consumed between 300 and 400 oz.; and 1 per cent of the Italians and 40 per cent of the Italian Americans consumed more than 400 oz.

Table 23.—*Weekly Consumption of Total Fluids in Ounces (in Per Cent)*

Italians				Italian Americans				
Male	*Female*	*Total*		*Male*		*Female*		*Total*
				1st	2d+3d	1st	2d+3d	
(*N*=*125*)	(*N*=*122*)	(*N*=*247*)		(*N*=*28*)	(*N*=*81*)	(*N*=*44*)	(*N*=*98*)	(*N*=*251*)
14	15	14	0–100	0	0	0	0	0
36	59	47	101–200	4	2	9	4	4
40	23	31	201–300	29	10	30	33	24
8	3	6	301–400	25	27	27	42	32
2	0	1	401–500	25	26	25	15	22
0	0	0	501–600	4	19	5	4	9
0	0	0	601–700	11	11	2	1	6
0	0	0	701–800	3	1	0	0	1
0	0	0	801–900	0	2	0	0	1
0	0	0	901–1,000	0	1	0	1	1
0	0	0	No information	0	0	2	0	0
100	*100*	*99*	*Totals*	*101*	*99*	*100*	*100*	*100*

This is apparently the first time that such an observation has been made, and the meaning of the data cannot be overemphasized.

Among the Italians, who have a low incidence of alcoholism (8), the ingestion of total fluids is also low. Among the Italian Americans—a group in contact with a new culture and acquiring the habits of that culture—the ingestion of total fluids increases markedly from the first to the second and third generations among both men and women. Paralleling this increasing fluid ingestion, it will be noted later, is an increase of sporadic excessive drinking among Italian Americans. Moreover, another investigation[1] has indicated an increase in the incidence of alcoholism among Italian Americans, especially in the second and third generations.

Still another study,[1] conducted on known alcoholics, seems to indicate that these pathological drinkers of alcoholic beverages are also excessive drinkers of fluids in general. In some cases, before the onset of excessive drinking of alcohol, excessive drinking of fluids had been common.

All these findings tend to show that alcoholics are excessive drinkers of fluids before becoming alcoholics, and to corroborate the view that alcoholism is an extreme deviation of a normal drinking habit.

Water

During the week of observation, as shown in Table 24, 14 per cent of the Italians—22 per cent of the men and 6 per cent of the women—drank no water at all. Their need for liquids was satisfied by other fluids, in most cases wine. Among the Italian Americans, 7 per cent of both the men and the women consumed no water.

Only 10 per cent of the Italians but 26 per cent of the Italian Americans drank between 129 and 256 oz. of water during the week, while 2 per cent of the Italians and 5 per cent of the Italian Americans drank more than 256 oz.

Milk

The use of milk, like that of water, was found to be strikingly higher among the Italian-American subjects. As shown in Table 25, 14 per cent of the Italians—11 per cent of the men and 17

[1] LOLLI, G. Unpublished observation, Yale Plan Clinic, New Haven, Conn., and Knickerbocker Hospital, New York City.

TABLE 24.—*Weekly Consumption of Water in Ounces (in Per Cent)*

Italians				Italian Americans				
Male	*Female*	*Total*		*Male*		*Female*		*Total*
				1st	2d+3d	1st	2d+3d	
(*N*=*125*)	(*N*=*122*)	(*N*=*247*)		(*N*=*28*)	(*N*=*81*)	(*N*=*44*)	(*N*=*98*)	(*N*=*251*)
22	6	14	None	14	5	9	6	7
2	1	1	1–4	0	0	0	0	0
3	1	2	5–8	0	4	0	1	2
4	1	2	9–16	0	2	0	8	4
3	7	5	17–32	7	7	14	14	11
23	25	24	33–64	21	14	27	14	17
26	53	39	65–128	18	31	18	31	27
14	6	10	129–256	32	31	23	22	26
3	1	2	257 or more	7	6	7	3	5
0	0	0	No information	0	0	2	0	0
100	*101*	*99*	*Totals*	*99*	*100*	*100*	*99*	*99*

TABLE 25.–*Weekly Consumption of Milk in Ounces (in Per Cent)*

ITALIANS				ITALIAN AMERICANS				
Male	*Female*	*Total*		*Male*		*Female*		*Total*
				1st	2d+3d	1st	2d+3d	
(N=125)	(N=122)	(N=247)		(N=28)	(N=81)	(N=44)	(N=98)	(N=251)
11	17	14	None	11	0	2	3	3
4	7	5	1–4	7	0	2	2	2
6	2	4	5–8	7	1	5	4	3
11	7	10	9–16	14	5	16	8	9
23	21	22	17–32	18	17	11	20	18
23	27	25	33–64	14	31	27	33	29
20	16	18	65–128	21	33	25	23	26
2	2	2	129–256	7	10	9	6	8
0	0	0	257 or more	0	2	0	0	1
0	0	0	No information	0	0	2	0	0
100	*99*	*100*	*Totals*	*99*	*99*	*99*	*99*	*99*

per cent of the women—but only 3 per cent of the Italian Americans drank no milk during the period of observation. A small quantity, between 1 and 8 oz. per week, was consumed by 9 per cent of the Italians and 5 per cent of the Italian Americans, usually in combination with coffee.

Quantities of 33 to 64 oz. (5 to 8 glasses) were consumed by 25 per cent of the Italians and 29 per cent of the Italian Americans, while 65 to 128 ounces (about 9 to 16 glasses) were consumed by 18 per cent of the Italians and 26 per cent of the Italian Americans. Only 2 per cent of the Italians but 9 per cent of the Italian Americans drank more than 16 glasses of milk weekly.

There is, therefore, no doubt that the consumption of milk is higher among adult Italian Americans than among adult Italians[2] —a trend which parallels a decrease in breast-feeding experiences in the Italian-American group. The full physiological and psychological significance of this higher milk consumption, however, is not clear. Although it has been suggested that the consumption of milk might be an index of the nutritional standards of a civilization, the broad implications of such an assumption may be questioned. It should be noted that high nutritional standards and prevention of illness are not one and the same thing. In countries where there is a high adult consumption of milk, there is also a high consumption of fats, with possibly dangerous effects on the cardiovascular system.

Accordingly, while the nutritional value of whole milk as food for the infant remains unchallenged, its nutritional value as food for the adult is at least not unlimited.

"Soft" Drinks[3]

During the week of observation, 96 per cent of the Italians consumed no "soft drinks" whatsoever, and 2 per cent consumed less than 9 oz.

On the other hand, nearly three-quarters of the Italian Americans drank these beverages, often in considerable amounts. As shown in Table 26, 15 per cent of these subjects used 1 or 2 glasses (9 to 16 oz.) during the week of record, 16 per cent used 2 to 4 glasses,

[2] The findings on adult Italians agree with those in a survey of a stratified sample of the population of Italy. Cf. Part II.

[3] "Soft drinks" include the popular sweetened as well as unsweetened and usually carbonated beverages, but not fruit juices, milk or water.

TABLE 26.—*Weekly Consumption of Soft Drinks in Ounces (in Per Cent)*

Italians: Male	Italians: Female	Italians: Total		Italian Americans: Male 1st	Italian Americans: Male 2d+3d	Italian Americans: Female 1st	Italian Americans: Female 2d+3d	Italian Americans: Total
(*N*=*125*)	(*N*=*122*)	(*N*=*247*)		(*N*=*28*)	(*N*=*81*)	(*N*=*44*)	(*N*=*98*)	(*N*=*251*)
95	98	96	None	61	19	39	22	28
3	0	2	1–4	0	1	0	3	2
1	0	0	5–8	7	6	9	19	12
0	0	0	9–16	7	12	9	24	15
1	2	1	17–32	4	20	25	13	16
0	0	0	33–64	4	22	14	15	16
0	0	0	65–128	14	20	2	2	9
0	0	0	129–256	4	0	0	1	1
0	0	0	No information	0	0	2	0	0
100	*100*	*99*	*Totals*	*101*	*100*	*100*	*99*	*99*

TABLE 27.—*Weekly Consumption of Fruit Juices in Ounces (in Per Cent)*

Italians: Male	Italians: Female	Italians: Total		Italian Americans: Male 1st	Italian Americans: Male 2d+3d	Italian Americans: Female 1st	Italian Americans: Female 2d+3d	Italian Americans: Total
(*N*=*125*)	(*N*=*122*)	(*N*=*247*)		(*N*=*28*)	(*N*=*81*)	(*N*=*44*)	(*N*=*98*)	(*N*=*251*)
86	89	86	None	50	43	48	20	36
9	7	8	1–4	4	5	5	4	4
4	1	2	5–8	7	2	7	7	6
1	2	2	9–16	14	9	11	16	13
1	1	1	17–32	14	26	18	31	25
0	0	0	33–64	11	14	5	16	13
0	0	0	65–128	0	1	5	5	3
0	0	0	No information	0	0	2	0	0
101	*100*	*99*	*Totals*	*100*	*100*	*101*	*99*	*100*

16 per cent used 4 to 8 glasses, and 9 per cent used 8 to 16 glasses. In this group, it is obvious, "soft drinks" contributed significantly to the caloric intake of the subjects.

Fruit Juices

Analysis of the use of fruit juices, as indicated in Table 27, likewise shows striking differences between the Italian and Italian-American subjects.

Only 13 per cent of the Italians drank any juice during the week, and only 2 subjects drank as much as 17 to 32 oz. In marked contrast, 64 per cent of the Italian Americans drank fruit juice and 41 per cent consumed more than 17 oz. per week.

Coffee

The data on the ingestion of coffee, given in Table 28, are not entirely comparable for the two groups. Because of differences in roasting and packing, the same amount of coffee yields in the United States a fluid volume which is double that yielded in Italy. Although the stimulant values of coffee in the two countries therefore cannot be compared directly, it is possible to consider the volumes of liquid involved and the contributions of these volumes to the total fluid intake of the subjects. On this basis it is evident that again the consumption of the Italian Americans was significantly larger than that of the Italians.

During the week of observation, 78 per cent of the Italians used coffee, but none of these subjects consumed more than 96 oz. Among the Italian Americans, 97 per cent took coffee; 40 per cent drank 97 to 180 oz., 13 per cent drank 181 to 240 oz., and 9 per cent drank more than 240 oz., i.e., more than 4 cups a day.

Alcoholic Beverages

Wine

The consistent and considerable use of wine as a beverage among the Italian subjects is illustrated in Table 29, as is the progressive decrease in its use among the Italian-American subjects.

During the week of observation, only 10 per cent of the Italian men but 32 per cent of the first-generation and 53 per cent of the second- and third-generation men in the Italian-American group abstained from wine entirely. This trend was even more obvious among the female subjects. Complete abstention from wine was

TABLE 28.–*Weekly Consumption of Coffee in Ounces (in Per Cent)*

Italians				Italian Americans				
Male	*Female*	*Total*		*Male*		*Female*		*Total*
				1st	2d+3d	1st	2d+3d	
(*N*=*125*)	(*N*=*122*)	(*N*=*247*)		(*N*=*28*)	(*N*=*81*)	(*N*=*44*)	(*N*=*98*)	(*N*=*251*)
33	11	22	None	4	1	2	4	3
11	16	14	1–6	0	0	0	0	0
38	47	42	7–18	0	1	2	3	2
10	19	14	19–30	4	0	2	0	1
6	6	6	31–48	11	4	7	5	6
2	2	2	49–96	21	26	25	30	26
0	0	0	97–180	54	36	43	38	40
0	0	0	181–240	7	17	7	14	13
0	0	0	241 or more	0	15	9	6	9
0	0	0	No information	0	0	2	0	0
100	*101*	*100*	*Totals*	*101*	*100*	*99*	*100*	*100*

TABLE 29.—*Weekly Consumption of Wine in Ounces*[1] *(in Per Cent)*

Italians				Italian Americans				
Male	*Female*	*Total*		*Male*		*Female*		*Total*
				1st	2d+3d	1st	2d+3d	
(*N*=*125*)	(*N*=*122*)	(*N*=*247*)		(*N*=*28*)	(*N*=*81*)	(*N*=*44*)	(*N*=*98*)	(*N*=*251*)
10	24	17	None	32	53	48	66	55
2	5	3	1–4	0	7	9	10	8
4	4	4	5–8	7	11	2	6	7
4	10	7	9–16	7	6	11	9	8
10	19	14	17–32	14	12	11	4	9
19	30	25	33–64	18	8	14	4	8
38	7	22	65–128	18	1	2	0	3
11	1	6	129–256	0	1	0	0	0
2	0	1	257 or more	4	0	0	0	0
0	0	0	No information	0	0	2	0	0
100	*100*	99	*Totals*	*100*	99	99	99	98

[1] For calculation of the consumption of absolute alcohol the wines included here may be taken at 10 per cent by volume.

reported by 24 per cent of the Italian women and 48 per cent of the first-generation and 66 per cent of the second- and third-generation women among the Italian Americans. It will be noted later, however, that none of the Italians and very few of the Italian Americans abstained consistently from all alcoholic beverages.

Nevertheless, it is clear that there is not only a trend away from the use of wine by Italian Americans, but also that sex differences in the use of wine—differences which are particularly obvious in Italy—tend to disappear when Italians migrate to the United States.

The ingestion of 65 to 256 oz. of wine per week, approximately between 2 and 9 glasses of wine per day, was reported by 49 per cent of the Italian men and 8 per cent of the Italian women. Most of the Italian women drank at least 1 glass per week but not more than 2 glasses per day. The record of the Italian Americans is strikingly different. Only 18 per cent of the first-generation men and 2 per cent of the second- and third-generation men drank from 2 to 8 glasses daily. Only 1 Italian-American woman reported the use of such quantities.

Beer

As shown in Table 30, the consumption of beer was negligible in the Italian group. No beer at all was used during the week by 85 per cent of the Italian men and 90 per cent of the women, and 6 per cent of the men and 8 per cent of the women consumed no more than 12 oz. in that period.

In contrast, among the Italian Americans, beer was used by 46 per cent of the men and 40 per cent of the women in the first-generation group, and by 70 per cent of the men and 37 per cent of the women in the second- and third-generation group. Approximately 36 per cent of the Italian Americans drank more than 12 oz. of beer during the week.

Aperitifs

Analysis of the use of aperitifs showed no significant differences between the Italians and the Italian Americans. The overwhelming majority—88 per cent of the Italians and 90 per cent of the Italian-Americans—used none of these beverages during the week, while 11 per cent of the Italians and 6 per cent of the Italian Americans drank 2 oz. or less. Quantities of 3 to 10 oz. were consumed by 1 per cent of the Italians and 3 per cent of the Italian Americans.

TABLE 30.—*Weekly Consumption of Beer in Ounces*[1] *(in Per Cent)*

Italians				Italian Americans				
Male	*Female*	*Total*		*Male*		*Female*		*Total*
				1st	2d+3d	1st	2d+3d	
(*N*=*125*)	(*N*=*122*)	(*N*=*247*)		(*N*=*28*)	(*N*=*81*)	(*N*=*44*)	(*N*=*98*)	(*N*=*251*)
85	90	87	None	54	30	59	63	51
6	8	7	1–12	0	9	16	19	13
6	2	4	13–36	14	25	20	13	19
2	0	1	37–72	18	15	2	3	8
0	0	0	73–144	11	17	0	0	6
0	0	0	145 or more	4	5	0	1	2
0	0	0	No information	0	0	2	0	0
99	*100*	*99*	*Totals*	*99*	*101*	*99*	*99*	*99*

[1] For calculation of the consumption of absolute alcohol the beer may be taken at 4 per cent by volume.

TABLE 31.—*Weekly Consumption of Distilled Spirits in Ounces*[1] *(in Per Cent)*

Italians				Italian Americans				
Male	*Female*	*Total*		*Male*		*Female*		*Total*
				1st	2d+3d	1st	2d+3d	
(*N*=*125*)	(*N*=*122*)	(*N*=*247*)		(*N*=*28*)	(*N*=*81*)	(*N*=*44*)	(*N*=*98*)	(*N*=*251*)
94	99	96	None	67	46	70	67	61
2	1	2	1	4	10	11	11	10
2	0	1	2	4	6	0	10	6
1	0	0.5	3–5	7	14	16	8	11
1	0	0.5	6–10	14	12	0	2	6
0	0	0	11–20	4	12	0	0	4
0	0	0	21 or more	0	0	0	1	0
0	0	0	No information	0	0	2	0	0
100	*100*	*100*	*Totals*	*100*	*100*	99	99	98

[1] For calculation of the consumption of absolute alcohol the distilled spirits may be taken at 44 per cent alcohol by volume.

One man, a first-generation Italian American, reported drinking more than 20 oz. during the week.

Distilled Spirits

As shown in Table 31, distilled spirits in one form or another were used during the week by only 4 per cent of the Italians but 39 per cent of the Italian Americans.

In the Italian-American group, spirits were used by 33 per cent of the men and 29 per cent of the women among the first-generation subjects, and by 54 per cent of the men and 33 per cent of the women in the second- and third-generation group.

No Italian subject recorded the use of more than 10 oz. of distilled spirits during the week, while at least this amount was ingested by one first-generation Italian-American man and by 12 per cent of the men and 1 per cent of the women among the second- and third-generation subjects.

The marked abstention of the Italians and the low consumption of the Italian-American women stand in sharp contrast to the considerable and increasing use of distilled spirits by Italian-American men.

Total Alcoholic Beverages

The total volumes of alcoholic beverages used during the week of observation are summarized in Table 32.

While only 14 per cent of the Italian subjects used no alcoholic beverages at all, 23 per cent of the Italian Americans were abstainers during the week.

Alcoholic beverages in quantities of 65 to 256 oz. of fluid were consumed by 50 per cent of the Italian men, 10 per cent of the Italian women, 43 per cent of the first-generation Italian-American men, 5 per cent of the first-generation women, 32 per cent of the second- and third-generation men, and 2 per cent of the second- and third-generation women.

Thus, as noted earlier, the incidence of alcoholism among Italians is low and the volume of total fluids consumed is also low, as shown in Table 23, but the volume of total alcoholic beverages—mostly in the form of wine—is relatively high. In contrast, it appears that the Italian Americans consume relatively large volumes of total fluids but relatively small volumes of alcoholic beverages.

TABLE 32.—*Total Weekly Consumption of All Alcoholic Beverages in Ounces (in Per Cent)*

ITALIANS				ITALIAN AMERICANS				
Male	*Female*	*Total*		*Male*		*Female*		*Total*
				1st	2d+3d	1st	2d+3d	
(*N*=*125*)	(*N*=*122*)	(*N*=*247*)		(*N*=*28*)	(*N*=*81*)	(*N*=*44*)	(*N*=*98*)	(*N*=*251*)
6	21	14	None	14	16	20	34	23
3	7	5	1–4	0	2	11	17	10
4	6	5	5–8	7	2	5	7	6
5	8	6	9–16	4	6	14	15	11
10	19	14	17–32	18	20	25	14	18
19	29	24	33–64	11	21	18	10	15
39	9	24	65–128	18	17	5	1	9
11	1	6	129–256	25	15	0	1	8
2	0	1	257 or more	4	0	0	0	0
0	0	0	No information	0	0	2	0	0
99	*100*	*99*	*Totals*	*101*	*99*	*100*	*99*	*100*

Alcohol Content of Beverages

The ethyl alcohol content of the table wines, aperitifs, beer and distilled spirits consumed by the subjects is fairly constant for each of these classes of beverages and is shown in the footnotes to Tables 29, 30, and 31. It was therefore possible to determine with reasonable exactitude the total amounts of absolute alcohol consumed by these subjects, and these totals were taken into account in calculating the caloric values of the diets. By far the largest contributor of alcohol is wine, the traditional alcoholic beverage of the Italians, though this is almost entirely of the low-alcohol table-wine variety. Keller and Efron (10) calculated that in one year the absolute alcohol consumed in Italy was 11.07 liters per capita of the population aged 14 years and older. Of this, 10.4 l. (93 per cent) was from wine, only 0.47 l. from distilled spirits and only 0.21 l. from beer.

Caloric Value of Alcoholic Beverages

From the ethyl alcohol content of the alcoholic beverages, their caloric equivalents and the contribution of these alcohol calories to the total daily caloric intake of the subjects can be calculated.

The caloric significance of their wine consumption is indicated in Table 33. It is evident that wine represented 10 per cent or more of the total daily caloric intake for 37 per cent of the men and 6 per cent of the women among the Italians, for 19 per cent of the men and none of the women in the first-generation Italian-American group, and for 1 per cent of the men and none of the women in the second- and third-generation group.

These data provide additional evidence that, under the impact of a new culture, wine seems to lose its attraction and its significance as a fundamental part of the daily meal of the Italian-American subjects.

A similar analysis of the consumption of beer, summarized in Table 34, demonstrates that this beverage played a relatively minor part as a caloric source for the Italian subjects, but an increasingly important role for the Italian Americans.

The increasing importance of distilled spirits as a caloric source for the Italian-American subjects is shown in Table 35.

When the relationship of all alcoholic beverages is considered, as shown in Table 36, it is still obvious that alcohol supplied a larger portion of the total daily caloric intake for Italians than it

TABLE 33.–*Relation of Wine Calories to Total Daily Caloric Intake (in Per Cent)*

ITALIANS			*Per Cent of Total Intake*	ITALIAN AMERICANS				
Male	*Female*	*Total*		*Male*		*Female*		*Total*
(N=125)	(N=122)	(N=247)		1st (N=28)	2d+3d (N=81)	1st (N=44)	2d+3d (N=98)	(N=251)
10	24	17	None	32	53	48	63	55
4	7	6	Less than 1	4	11	9	11	10
10	15	12	1–2	11	17	9	13	14
19	22	21	3–5	21	14	16	6	12
21	26	23	6–9	14	4	16	3	6
24	3	14	10–14	11	0	0	0	1
9	2	6	15–19	4	1	0	0	1
2	1	1	20–24	0	0	0	0	0
2	0	1	25 or more	4	0	0	0	0
0	0	0	No information	0	0	2	0	0
101	*100*	*101*	*Totals*	*101*	*100*	*100*	*99*	*100*

TABLE 34.—*Relation of Beer Calories to Total Daily Caloric Intake (in Per Cent)*

Italians				Italian Americans				
Male	*Female*	*Total*	*Per Cent of Total Intake*	*Male*		*Female*		*Total*
				1st	2d+3d	1st	2d+3d	
(*N*=*125*)	(*N*=*122*)	(*N*=*247*)		(*N*=28)	(*N*=*81*)	(*N*=*44*)	(*N*=*98*)	(*N*=*251*)
85	90	86	None	54	30	59	63	51
8	7	8	Less than 1	0	10	9	13	10
5	2	3	1–2	11	25	23	16	19
2	1	2	3–5	21	21	5	6	12
0	0	0	6–9	11	14	2	0	6
0	0	0	10 or more	4	1	0	1	1
0	0	0	No information	0	0	2	0	0
100	*100*	*99*	*Totals*	*101*	*101*	*100*	*99*	*99*

TABLE 35.—*Relation of Distilled Spirits Calories to Total Daily Caloric Intake (in Per Cent)*

Italians				Italian Americans				
Male	*Female*	*Total*	*Per Cent of Total Intake*	*Male*		*Female*		*Total*
				1st	2d+3d	1st	2d+3d	
(*N*=*125*)	(*N*=*122*)	(*N*=*247*)		(*N*=28)	(*N*=*81*)	(*N*=*44*)	(*N*=*98*)	(*N*=*251*)
94	99	97	None	67	46	70	67	61
3	1	2	Less than 1	4	16	11	16	14
2	0	1	1–2	11	16	14	13	14
0	0	0	3–5	18	22	2	2	10
1	0	0	6 or more	0	0	0	1	0
0	0	0	No information	0	0	2	0	0
100	*100*	*100*	*Totals*	*100*	*100*	*99*	*99*	*99*

TABLE 36.—*Relation of Total Alcoholic Beverage Calories to Total Daily Caloric Intake (in Per Cent)*

ITALIANS				ITALIAN AMERICANS				
Male	*Female*	*Total*	*Per Cent of Total Intake*	*Male*		*Female*		*Total*
				1st	2d+3d	1st	2d+3d	
(*N*=*125*)	(*N*=*122*)	(*N*=*247*)		(*N*=*28*)	(*N*=*81*)	(*N*=*44*)	(*N*=*98*)	(*N*=*251*)
6	21	14	None	14	16	20	34	23
6	7	6	Less than 1	0	4	9	15	9
10	14	12	1–2	14	17	18	25	20
18	25	21	3–5	14	28	27	20	23
22	27	25	6–9	18	22	18	3	14
26	2	14	10–14	25	9	5	1	6
9	2	6	15–19	7	2	0	0	2
2	2	2	20–24	4	1	0	2	2
2	0	1	25 or more	4	0	0	0	0
0	0	0	No information	0	0	2	0	0
101	*100*	*101*	*Totals*	*100*	*99*	*99*	*100*	*99*

did for Italian Americans. Even though the latter demonstrated an increasing proclivity toward the use of beer and distilled spirits, this did not compensate for the greater use of wine by the Italian subjects.

Thus, it will be noted that all alcoholic beverages together provided 10 per cent or more of the total caloric intake for 39 per cent of the men and 6 per cent of the women among the Italians, but for only 19 per cent of the men and 4 per cent of the women among the Italian Americans.

It is interesting to note that LeBreton and Trémolières (12), on the basis of a survey by the Institut National d'Hygiène, estimated that in France between 10 and 15 per cent of the caloric intake of men is contributed by alcohol. For women the corresponding value is between 6 and 9 per cent. In the U.S.A., on the other hand, Jellinek (9) has calculated that "for nearly 54 per cent of the population ethyl alcohol is not a source of calories." For actual consumers of alcohol he estimated a daily average contribution of 190 calories per capita, which would be less than 8 per cent. However, men obtained three times as many calories from alcohol as women. Jellinek also calculated, based on the survey by Luzzatto-Fegiz (22), that in Italy 10 per cent of the male drinkers derive as much as 1,600 calories a day from wine.[4]

Geographical Origin and Alcohol Consumption

The proportion of wine in the daily diet was found to be highest among Italian men of Central extraction, with a mean value of 9.13±0.98 per cent of the total daily caloric intake. Mean values for those of Northern and Southern origin were 5.80±0.86 and 6.78±0.84 per cent, respectively.

For Italian women, the mean values were 5.67±1.06 per cent for those of Central extraction, 3.07±0.41 per cent for those of Northern extraction, and 3.64±0.55 per cent for those of Southern extraction.

Among the Italian Americans, the mean values were highest for those of Northern and Central origin, and lowest for those of Southern extraction.

Analysis of the consumption of all alcoholic beverages indicated that these supplied the highest proportion of the total daily caloric intake among Italian men and women of Central origin.

[4] For a thorough analysis of the caloric contribution of alcohol to the adult population in Italy, see Part II.

Chapter 5

DRINKING HABITS

AN UNDERSTANDING of the present use of alcohol and the drinking behavior of adults depends at least in part on an understanding of the early drinking experiences of these individuals. Accordingly, in this investigation, the early exposures of the subjects to alcoholic beverages were analyzed, together with their present drinking habits and attitudes, the relationships between their eating and drinking, and the occurrence of alcohol intoxication.

Earliest Drinking Experiences

The age at which the subjects first tasted an alcoholic beverage—though not necessarily drank it in any considerable amount—is indicated in Table 37.

Although some subjects were unable to recall their earliest experience, only one subject—a woman in the second- and third-generation Italian-American group—reported never having tasted alcohol. The exposure of all the other subjects to alcohol is presumably due to the fact that they were drawn from a population which has no prohibitions against alcoholic beverages. In such a population there are practically no fears attendant upon the drinking of alcohol, and the experience is so widespread as to represent a fact of life of almost the same import as the use of bread.

The data in Table 37 appear to be of extreme importance. It is evident that 61 per cent of the Italian men and 58 per cent of the Italian women tasted an alcoholic beverage before reaching their eleventh birthday, as did 79 per cent of the men and 87 per cent of the women among the first-generation Italian Americans, and 72 per cent of the men and 80 per cent of the women in the second- and third-generation group. A further analysis shows that a considerable number of Italians were exposed to an alcoholic beverage between the ages of 2 and 5, as were many in both the Italian-American groups.

It is also interesting to note that only small proportions of the various groups—18 per cent of the Italians and 3 per cent of the Italian Americans—were unable to give information about these

TABLE 37.—*Age (Years) at First Taste of Alcoholic Beverage (in Per Cent)*

ITALIANS				ITALIAN AMERICANS				
Male	*Female*	*Total*		*Male*		*Female*		*Total*
				1st	2d+3d	1st	2d+3d	
(*N*=*125*)	(*N*=*122*)	(*N*=*247*)		(*N*=*28*)	(*N*=*81*)	(*N*=*44*)	(*N*=*98*)	(*N*=*251*)
0	0	0	Never drank	0	0	0	1	0
1	1	1	Less than ½	4	2	0	2	2
2	2	2	½–2	11	16	32	25	22
21	13	17	2–5	39	23	32	19	25
37	42	39	6–10	25	31	23	33	30
18	11	14	11–15	14	15	7	9	11
8	7	8	16–20	7	9	2	6	6
0	1	0	21 or over	0	0	0	1	0
14	24	18	No information	0	4	5	3	3
101	*101*	99	*Totals*	*100*	*100*	*101*	99	99

early drinking experiences. It was observed time and again during this inquiry that the Italians and even more the Italian Americans had vivid recollections of past events in their own lives and in their families. In the case of the Italian Americans it is as though, in contact with a new culture which challenged their old standards, they constantly tried to cast light on their past history and to examine facts and events in order to acquire from them the strength necessary for consistent behavior. By and large, this awareness of early drinking experiences duplicates the awareness of early feeding experiences described previously.

The type of beverage involved in these first tasting experiences is shown in Table 38. This beverage was wine for 91 per cent of the Italians, 93 per cent of the first-generation Italian Americans, and 85 per cent of the second- and third-generation Italian Americans.

The occasion of the first drinking experience is shown in Table 39. Here a significant difference is evident between Italians and Americans of Italian extraction. While 83 per cent of the Italians considered their first exposure to alcohol as part of their regular family, social or religious life, only 8 per cent of the Italian Americans offered this explanation and 75 per cent of them interpreted their first use of an alcoholic beverage as a "casual sip-taste." In this connection, however, it must be emphasized that this interpretation of early drinking experiences by the Italian-American subjects might have been colored by beliefs and standards drawn from a new environment. It must also be emphasized again that these Americans of Italian extraction do not necessarily represent all Italian Americans in the United States.

Present Drinking Patterns

Information on the alcoholic beverages now used by the subjects, as shown in Table 40, was obtained from the dietary records as amplified by statements made by the subjects.

Wine is the only type of alcoholic beverage used by the great majority of Italians. It is the exclusive beverage of 63 per cent of the men and 70 per cent of the women. On the other hand, wine is used exclusively by only 4 per cent of the first-generation and 2 per cent of the second- and third-generation Italian Americans.

The more frequent use of alcoholic beverages other than wine by the Italian Americans may be attributed to availability of these other beverages and to a variety of psychosocial factors. It is highly

TABLE 38.–*Beverages Used in First Tasting Experience (in Per Cent)*

Italians: *Male*	Italians: *Female*	Italians: *Total*		Italian Americans: *Male* 1st	Italian Americans: *Male* 2d+3d	Italian Americans: *Female* 1st	Italian Americans: *Female* 2d+3d	Italian Americans: *Total*
(*N*=125)	(*N*=122)	(*N*=247)		(*N*=28)	(*N*=81)	(*N*=44)	(*N*=98)	(*N*=251)
0	0	0	Never drank	0	0	0	1	0
1	2	2	Beer	0	5	2	6	4
91	93	91	Wine	96	86	91	83	87
0	0	0	Aperitif	0	0	2	1	1
4	2	3	Distilled spirits	0	2	0	5	3
1	0	0	Combination	0	2	0	1	1
3	2	3	No information	4	4	5	2	3
100	*99*	*99*	*Totals*	*100*	*99*	*100*	*99*	*99*

TABLE 39.–*Occasion of First Drinking Experience (in Per Cent)*

Italians: *Male*	Italians: *Female*	Italians: *Total*		Italian Americans: *Male* 1st	Italian Americans: *Male* 2d+3d	Italian Americans: *Female* 1st	Italian Americans: *Female* 2d+3d	Italian Americans: *Total*
(*N*=125)	(*N*=122)	(*N*=247)		(*N*=28)	(*N*=81)	(*N*=44)	(*N*=98)	(*N*=251)
0	0	0	None	0	0	0	1	0
2	1	1	Casual sip-taste	75	67	80	79	75
5	0	2	Experiment, joke	7	11	0	2	5
0	0	0	Medicine	4	1	5	4	3
8	6	7	Special occasion	7	10	7	3	6
78	89	83	Part of regular family, social or religious custom	7	9	5	8	8
8	5	6	No information	0	2	4	2	2
101	*101*	*99*	*Totals*	*100*	*100*	*101*	*99*	*99*

TABLE 40.—*Beverages Used in Present Drinking (in Per Cent)*

Italians Male	Italians Female	Italians Total		Italian Americans Male		Italian Americans Female		Italian Americans Total
				1st	2d+3d	1st	2d+3d	
(N=125)	(N=122)	(N=247)		(N=28)	(N=81)	(N=44)	(N=98)	(N=251)
0	0	0	None	4	5	5	4	4
63	70	66	Wine (W)	4	1	0	2	2
2	2	2	Beer (B)	0	0	2	0	0
0	0	0	Aperitif (A)	0	0	2	0	0
1	3	2	Distilled spirits (D)	0	1	2	4	2
10	8	9	W and B	7	1	7	1	3
3	7	5	W and A	7	0	7	1	2
10	2	6	W and D	4	1	5	2	2
0	0	0	B and A	0	0	0	0	0
0	1	0	B and D	4	4	0	5	4
0	0	0	A and D	0	0	2	1	1
1	2	2	W, B and A	0	1	2	2	2
3	2	2	W, B and D	21	30	9	18	21
6	1	3	W, A and D	4	1	2	8	5
0	0	0	B, A and D	0	6	2	2	3
2	1	2	W, B, A and D	46	47	48	49	48
0	0	0	No information	0	1	5	0	1
101	*99*	*99*	*Totals*	*101*	*99*	*100*	*99*	*100*

possible that, as in many other minority groups, the rejection of food habits which are part of their original culture is part of the rejection of the country of origin. For some Italian Americans, wine may be too closely identified with their country of origin. Whatever the reasons, wine has ceased to be the almost exclusive alcoholic beverage of Italians transplanted to the American culture.

Only 2 per cent of the Italians and less than 1 per cent of the Italian Americans now use beer exclusively, while distilled spirits are used exclusively by 2 per cent of the Italians and 2 per cent of the Italian Americans.

Both beer and wine are used by 9 per cent of the Italians and 3 per cent of the Italian Americans. A combined use of distilled spirits and wine was reported by 10 per cent of the men and 2 per cent of the women among the Italians, and by 2 per cent of the men and 3 per cent of the women among the Italian Americans. A combination of wine, beer and spirits is now used by 2 per cent of the Italians and 21 per cent of the Italian Americans. Use of a combination of wine, beer, spirits and aperitifs was listed by 2 per cent of the Italians and 48 per cent of the Italian Americans.

Significantly, the use of all four beverages was reported by essentially the same proportions of men and women—46 per cent of the men and 48 per cent of the women in the first-generation group of Italian Americans, and 47 per cent of the men and 49 per cent of the women in the second- and third-generation group. In terms of variety of choice of alcoholic beverages, it appears that differences between the sexes are nonexistent among Italian Americans.

The Italians and the Italian Americans gave quite different explanations of their present use of alcoholic beverages. A summary of their "reasons" is presented in Table 41.

One of the most striking differences concerned the reason of "sociability," or facilitating social intercourse, which in both lay and professional circles is repeatedly listed as one of the main functions of alcohol (5). This reason was given by less than 1 per cent of the Italians, but by 18 per cent of the men and 32 per cent of the women in the first-generation Italian-American group, and 41 per cent of the men and 44 per cent of the women in the second- and third-generation group. It is again evident that, among the Italian-American subjects, sex differences in attitudes toward alcoholic beverages tend to disappear. It is also evident that, among

TABLE 41.—*Reasons for Present Drinking (in Per Cent)*

Italians: *Male*	Italians: *Female*	Italians: *Total*		Italian Americans: *Male* 1st	Italian Americans: *Male* 2d+3d	Italian Americans: *Female* 1st	Italian Americans: *Female* 2d+3d	Italian Americans: *Total*
(*N*=*125*)	(*N*=*122*)	(*N*=*247*)		(*N*=*28*)	(*N*=*81*)	(*N*=*44*)	(*N*=*98*)	(*N*=*251*)
1	1	1	Sociability	18	41	32	44	38
2	1	2	Likes taste	14	4	11	13	10
0	0	0	Sociability and taste	7	14	2	15	11
20	19	19	Health	14	1	9	0	4
27	39	33	Likes to drink	4	16	7	7	10
18	8	13	Health and likes to drink	18	5	14	1	6
2	2	2	Celebrate	0	1	0	0	0
15	20	18	Tradition	0	0	2	1	1
12	1	6	Effect	4	5	5	8	6
2	8	5	Medicinal	0	0	7	0	1
0	1	0	No reason or no information	18	9	7	6	8
0	0	0	Does not drink	4	5	5	4	4
99	*100*	*99*	*Totals*	*101*	*101*	*101*	*99*	*99*

the Italian subjects, other reasons than socializing predominate in the conscious motivation of drinking alcoholic beverages.

The reason given most commonly by the Italian subjects was that they like to drink—an explanation believed to be more inclusive than merely to like the taste of an alcoholic beverage. This attitude was expressed by 33 per cent of the Italians but only 10 per cent of the Italian Americans.

Another major reason, given by 19 per cent of the Italians, was based on drinking for health. This reflects the deeply rooted belief among Italians that wine used in moderation is a healthful constituent of the diet (31).[1] This belief seems to be disappearing among Italian Americans, with only 11 per cent of the first-generation and less than 1 per cent of the second- and third-generation subjects declaring that they drink for reasons of health.

The broad reason of "tradition" was given by 18 per cent of the Italians and less than 1 per cent (two women) of the Italian Americans.

"Effect" was presented as the main reason for drinking by 12 per cent of the men and 1 per cent of the women among the Italian subjects, 4 per cent of the men and 5 per cent of the women among the first-generation Italian Americans, and 5 per cent of the men and 8 per cent of the women among the second- and third-generation group. Here the interesting finding seems to be an increase of drinking for "effect" observed in Italian-American women.

It is not assumed that the "reasons" cited by the subjects necessarily represent the true or only motivations underlying the behavior of drinking alcoholic beverages. The Italian subjects who, in the roles of host and guest, drink a glass of wine together, might assign health (because of the accompanying toast) or tradition as the reason for drinking on that occasion. American subjects of Italian extraction might assign sociability as the reason for the same behavior on the like occasion. Nevertheless, the conscious choice to assign one reason or another reflects basic attitudes toward the use of alcoholic beverages, and it is clear from the choice expressed by the Italian-American subjects that they have moved toward the attitude more common among other American populations—that drinking is for the purpose of facilitating social intercourse.

[1] Cf. also Part II.

Drinking Patterns in Relation to Meals

Among the most significant findings obtained in this project are those concerned with the drinking patterns of the subjects in relation to their meals.

As shown in Table 42, only one subject—a first-generation Italian-American woman—reported customarily drinking only before meals, which here means drinking not more than an hour prior to the ingestion of solid food at the regular meal time. Only 1 per cent of the Italians and 4 per cent of the Italian Americans drank exclusively after meals, which here means not later than 4 to 5 hours after a regular meal. While 1 per cent of the Italians drank exclusively between meals, none of the Italian Americans reported such a practice. A combination of drinking before, with, after and between meals was noted in 15 per cent of the Italians and 79 per cent of the Italian-Americans—71 per cent of the first-generation and 83 per cent of the second- and third-generation groups.

Most important, however, is the observation that 70 per cent of the men and 94 per cent of the women among the Italians drank exclusively with meals, at regular meal times. This is in contrast to 7 per cent of the men and 16 per cent of the women in the first-generation Italian-American group, and 4 per cent of the men and 11 per cent of the women in the second- and third-generation group.

Moreover, a further inspection of the data on the Italian group revealed that the exclusive use of alcoholic beverages with meals was associated with consumption of smaller quantities of alcohol. Of those men whose alcohol consumption represented less than 10 per cent of the total daily caloric intake, 74 per cent drank exclusively with meals. Of those whose alcohol consumption provided more than 10 per cent of the total caloric intake, 64 per cent drank exclusively with meals. Similarly, among the women with relatively low consumption of alcohol, 97 per cent drank exclusively with meals, while of those with a higher alcohol ingestion, only 57 per cent drank exclusively with meals.

It has already been shown that individuals who drink only with meals are best protected against possible untoward reactions resulting from the use of excessive amounts of alcohol (4). Many physiological reasons underlie this protection. When the stomach is filled with solid food, the absorption of ethyl alcohol into the blood stream is delayed; accordingly, blood alcohol concentrations

TABLE 42.—*Time of Drinking of Alcoholic Beverages in Relation to Meal Times (in Per Cent)*

ITALIANS				ITALIAN AMERICANS				
Male	*Female*	*Total*		*Male*		*Female*		*Total*
				1st	2d+3d	1st	2d+3d	
(*N*=*125*)	(*N*=*122*)	(*N*=*247*)		(*N*=*28*)	(*N*=*81*)	(*N*=*44*)	(*N*=*98*)	(*N*=*251*)
0	0	0	Before meals	0	0	2	0	0
70	94	82	With meals	7	4	16	11	9
1	2	1	After meals	11	4	0	4	4
2	1	1	Between meals	0	0	0	0	0
27	3	15	Combination	71	85	70	80	79
0	0	0	No information	11	7	11	4	7
100	*100*	99	*Totals*	*100*	*100*	99	99	99

are lower than those observed when the same amounts of alcohol are taken on an empty stomach. Furthermore, the ingestion of a meal—especially if it includes considerable amounts of slowly absorbable carbohydrates, as in the diet of Italians—prevents low or fluctuating blood sugar levels and thereby protects the central nervous system against some of the toxic effects of alcohol (3). Finally, there is experimental evidence that the rate of oxidation of alcohol is considerably faster when the alcohol is taken while the digestive processes are elicited by a meal (27). By speeding the elimination of the alcohol, this increase in oxidative rate likewise helps to prevent untoward physiological effects.

In addition to these physiological factors, there are other features which apparently contribute considerably to the value of drinking with rather than apart from meals. It should be noted that drinking with meals generally signifies an experience shared by members of a small and mutually controlling group—usually the family unit, where the interplay of male–female and adult–child relationships is of paramount importance. Thus, the shared use of an alcoholic beverage—which among the Italians means the shared use of wine—reflects a cohesion or "sociability" rather than a means to reach it.

The obvious disappearance of the habit of drinking wine exclusively with meals as observed among the Italian Americans deserves the most careful consideration. There seems to be little doubt that the custom of using alcoholic beverages separately from other food items is linked with a search for the psychological rather than the physiological effects of ethyl alcohol. As will be noted later, the trend away from drinking wine with meals may be linked with the increasing occurrence of alcohol intoxication among the Italian-American subjects.

Use of Wine and Regularity of Eating Pattern

In an effort to identify any possible relationship between the use of wine and either regular or sporadic eating habits, the subjects were divided according to whether they used wine in amounts representing more or less than 10 per cent of the total daily caloric intake.

Among the Italians, 67 men in the "less than 10 per cent" group could be divided into 79 per cent regular and 21 per cent sporadic eaters, while 45 men in the "more than 10 per cent" group could be divided into 80 per cent regular and 20 per cent sporadic eaters.

Of the 86 Italian women in the "less than 10 per cent" group, 85 per cent were regular and 15 per cent were sporadic eaters.

Of the first-generation Italian-American men, 13 belonged in the "less than 10 per cent" group and all were regular eaters. Five men in the "more than 10 per cent" group were described as 3 regular and 2 sporadic eaters. Of the 22 first-generation women, all in the "less than 10 per cent" group, 64 per cent were regular and 36 per cent were sporadic eaters.

Among the second- and third-generation subjects, 37 men in the "less than 10 per cent" group could be classified as 18 regular and 19 sporadic eaters. Of the 33 women, all in the "less than 10 per cent" group, 55 per cent were regular and 45 per cent were sporadic eaters.

As already indicated, sporadic eating patterns were found more frequently in the Italian-American subjects. From the data presented here, no link can be discerned between the development of such eating patterns and the use of large or small amounts of wine. Instead, the decreased incidence of regular eating habits among Italian Americans must be attributed to recently established cultural patterns.

Use of Alcoholic Beverages and Body Weight

The relationships between intake of alcoholic beverages and body weight have long been the basis of much discussion and have led to many contradictory statements. It often happens that uncontrolled drinkers, the real alcoholics, are underweight, while conversely it has been observed that some individuals who are heavy drinkers, if not real alcoholics, are overweight. Both phenomena can be understood if it is realized that alcohol is a calorie-yielding food which may be ingested at the expense of other foods or in addition to them.

This situation was apparent among the group of subjects studied here, especially among the Italian group.

Among the Italian men, 18 were 10 per cent or more underweight. The caloric contribution of alcoholic beverages—which consisted primarily of wine—to the total diet was between 10 and 14 per cent for 5 of these men and less than 10 per cent for the others.

Among the Italian men, also, 33 were 10 per cent or more overweight. In this group, the caloric contribution of wine to the total diet was less than 1 per cent for 2 men, 1 to 2 per cent for 2, 3 to

5 per cent for 8, 6 to 9 per cent for 5, 10 to 14 per cent for 7, 15 to 19 per cent for 6, 20 to 24 per cent for 2, and 25 to 29 per cent for 1.

From these data, and from similar findings in the underweight and overweight Italian women, it appears there is no substantial relationship between daily ingestion of alcoholic beverages and body weight.

Use of Alcoholic Beverages and Daily Caloric Intake

In order to determine whether or not a relationship exists between daily intake of alcoholic beverages and total caloric intake, a special analysis was made of the use of wine by the Italian subjects and their daily caloric consumption. For this purpose, the subjects were divided into "heavy eaters," who consumed 2,300 to 3,000 calories daily, "moderate eaters," 1,650 to 2,299 calories daily, and "light eaters," under 1,650 calories daily.[2]

Of the 67 Italian men who drank wine in amounts contributing less than 10 per cent to the daily caloric intake, 20 were classified as heavy eaters, 29 as moderate eaters, and 18 as light eaters. Of the 30 whose wine contributed 10 to 14 per cent of their daily caloric intake, 11 were heavy eaters, 17 were moderate eaters, and 2 were light eaters. On the other hand, of the 15 whose wine consumption represented 15 per cent or more of the daily caloric intake, 14 were heavy eaters and 1 was a moderate eater.

It appears that large amounts of wine were ingested together with large amounts of solid food, while the ingestion of small to moderate amounts of wine bore little or no relationship to light, moderate or heavy eating.

Approximately the same trend was noted among the Italian women. Of the 86 whose wine consumption contributed 10 per cent or less to the total daily caloric intake, 20 were classified as heavy eaters, 54 as moderate eaters, and 12 as light eaters. Of the 7 who drank wine in quantities representing 10 per cent or more of their daily caloric intake, 5 were heavy eaters and 2 moderate eaters.

Similarly, all the Italian Americans who drank wine in quantities representing 10 per cent or more of the daily caloric intake were classified as heavy eaters.

[2] Although sex, height, body frame and occupation should be taken into account in classifying eating habits for other purposes, the classification used here is adequate for the present inquiry.

Use of Wine in Relation to Use of Water and Milk

A comparison of the use of wine and of water among Italian subjects revealed an inverse relationship between consumption of these two beverages.

Among the men who drank wine in amounts representing less than 10 per cent of the total daily caloric intake, the amounts of water ingested during the week were as follows: none, 21 per cent; 1–16 oz. of water, 7 per cent; 17–64 oz., 29 per cent; and 65–256 oz., 43 per cent. Among the men whose wine consumption represented more than 10 per cent of the total caloric intake, the water consumption was: none, 29 per cent; 1–16 oz., 20 per cent; 17–64 oz., 25 per cent; and 65–256 oz., 27 per cent.

Among the Italian women whose wine consumption contributed less than 10 per cent to their total caloric intake, the water consumption during the week was: none, 4 per cent; 1–16 oz., none; 17–64 oz., 36 per cent; and 65–256 oz., 60 per cent. Among those with a wine consumption contributing more than 10 per cent to the total caloric intake, the water consumption was: none, 28 per cent; 1–16 oz., 28 per cent; 17–64 oz., 28 per cent; and 65–256 oz., 16 per cent.

On the other hand, no relationship was apparent between consumption of wine and consumption of milk. Among those Italian men whose use of wine represented less than 10 per cent and more than 10 per cent, respectively, of the total caloric intake, the consumption of milk during the week was as follows: none, 8 and 11 per cent; 1–16 oz., 24 and 22 per cent; 17–32 oz., 22 and 26 per cent; 33–64 oz., 24 and 20 per cent; and 65 oz. or more, 22 and 21 per cent.

Approximately the same percentages were noted among the Italian women who consumed wine in amounts contributing less than 10 per cent of the total caloric intake. Only seven Italian women used wine in large amounts. Of these, two drank no milk during the week, two drank less than 4 oz., two drank between 17 and 32 oz., and one drank more than 33 oz.

Of the first-generation Italian-American men who drank wine in quantities contributing less than 10 per cent of the total caloric intake, 1 drank no milk during the week, 10 drank less than 65 oz., and 3 drank more than 65 oz. Of those whose wine consumption was greater, 4 drank less than 65 oz. of milk and 1 drank more.

Use of Alcoholic Beverages in Relation to Diabetes

As part of the routine studies included in this project, glucose tolerance tests were performed in 476 of the subjects. After a fasting blood specimen was obtained, 50 g. of glucose dissolved in water was fed to each of the subjects, and capillary blood samples were then taken every half hour for 3 hours.

Glucose tolerance curves were considered normal if the peak was below 170 mg. per 100 cc. of blood and the curve fell to a fasting level (less than 120 mg. per 100 cc.) within 2 hours. The curves were considered diabetic if the peak was above 170 mg. per 100 cc. and the glucose concentration was more than 120 mg. per 100 cc. at 2 or 2½ hours after the administration of glucose. Curves which showed either a high peak or a delayed fall were considered borderline diabetic.

Altogether 58 borderline and 15 obviously diabetic glucose tolerance curves were found. Since none of the subjects had been aware of this abnormal condition, the discovery of the abnormal curve was accidental in every case.

It appears significant that most of these borderline or true diabetic subjects either drank no alcoholic beverages at all during the week of observation or consumed only very small quantities. Among the borderline cases, 14 subjects abstained, 29 consumed alcohol in amounts representing less than 10 per cent of the daily caloric intake, 10 drank alcohol in amounts representing from 10 to 19 per cent, and 5 consumed larger quantities. Among the diabetic subjects, 6 abstained, 7 consumed alcohol in amounts contributing less than 10 per cent to the total caloric intake, 1 drank amounts representing 10 to 19 per cent, and 1 drank larger amounts.

Only 1 of the diabetics and 20 of the borderline diabetics were found in the group of Italian subjects. The diabetic subject was an Italian male whose wine consumption contributed between 10 and 14 per cent of his daily caloric intake. Among the 12 Italian male borderline diabetics, 4 consumed wine in amounts representing 10 to 14 per cent of total caloric intake, while 2 drank more and 6 drank less. Among the 8 female borderline cases, 3 abstained, 4 drank wine in amounts corresponding to less than 10 per cent of the total caloric intake, and 1 in an amount corresponding to between 15 and 19 per cent.

Thus these diabetics and borderline cases were not constant regular users of wine.

It was noted later that excessive use of alcohol was relatively rare among these borderline or diabetic individuals. No instances of alcohol intoxication were reported by 23 of the 58 borderline cases and by 11 of the 15 diabetics. The occurrence of episodes of intoxication was reported by the borderline subjects as follows: 1 episode, 16; 2, 4; 3–4, 8; 5–9, 3; 10–14, 2; 15–19, 1; and 25 or more, 1. Among the diabetics, 2 subjects each reported 1 episode, 1 reported 2, and 1 reported 25 or more.

Conversely, when excessive use of alcohol was observed, signs of deranged carbohydrate metabolism were uncommon. Thus, all of the 11 Italian men who reported 25 or more episodes of intoxication were found to have a normal glucose tolerance. Among the Italian-American group, the glucose tolerance curves were normal in 11 and borderline in 1 of the 12 men who reported 25 or more episodes of intoxication and normal in all of the 4 women who described such numerous experiences.

Use of Alcoholic Beverages in Relation to Neurotic Traits[3]

During the prolonged disputes over the values and dangers of alcoholic beverages, there has been considerable controversy over the relationship between these beverages and various emotional illnesses. The alcohol consumption of those subjects who demonstrated any signs of emotional disorder was therefore analyzed separately.

None of the Italian subjects exhibited any psychotic traits. Only 21 (8.5 per cent) demonstrated signs of nonpsychotic emotional disorders ranging from minor emotional problems to anxieties arising from latent homosexuality. While some of these cases fell into the usual psychiatric classifications of anxiety hysteria, conversion hysteria, obsessions, compulsions and the like, most of them belonged to the ill-defined group of character neuroses.

Of the 16 Italian men with neurotic traits, 3 consumed alcoholic beverages in amounts representing 15 to 19 per cent of the total daily caloric intake, 12 drank amounts representing less than 14 per cent of the total intake, and 1 abstained entirely. Of the 5 Italian neurotic women, 2 abstained and 3 consumed amounts representing less than 9 per cent of the total caloric intake.

Among the Italian Americans, 13 men were classified as frank neurotics. Only 1 drank alcoholic beverages in amounts contributing

[3] An analysis of personality data in a portion of the Italian-American group has been presented in a separate report by Lisansky, Golder and Lolli (13).

as much as 10 to 14 per cent of the daily caloric intake, while 8 consumed smaller amounts and 4 abstained. Seven of these men drank no wine during the week of record, while the others drank it in amounts contributing less than 9 per cent of the total caloric intake.

The same pattern was observed among the 29 Italian-American women who were labeled as neurotics. Thirteen drank no alcoholic beverages during the week of observation, 15 consumed amounts representing less than 9 per cent of the total caloric intake, and 1 drank amounts representing between 20 and 24 per cent. Twenty of these women drank no wine during the observation period, and 9 consumed wine in amounts contributing less than 9 per cent of the total caloric intake.

In these groups there is no doubt that alcohol contributed but little to the development of neurotic traits. Further, when neurotic traits were present, they seldom or never led to the excessive and uncontrolled use of alcoholic beverages.

Use of Wine and Marital Status

Of the 13 Italian men who drank no wine during the week of observation, 10 were single while 3 were married and living with their wives. Of the 29 Italian women who drank no wine, 22 were single and 7 were married.

It would appear, therefore, that the use of wine—linked as it is with family events—loses much of its appeal for the unattached individual in the Italian culture, where alcoholic beverages are seldom used for "escape" purposes.

The situation among the Italian-American subjects was strikingly different. Of the 52 men who abstained from wine during the week, only 15 were single. Of the 87 women who abstained, only 17 were single.

It is not improbable that this finding reflects different meanings attached to alcoholic beverages in Italy and in the United States. This difference is considered in more detail in the following section.

Attitudes toward Drinking

Another important difference between the Italians and the Italian Americans was found in the attitudes expressed toward the use of alcoholic beverages.

Table 43 summarizes the attitudes of the fathers of the subjects

TABLE 43.—*Attitudes of Fathers of Subjects toward Use of Alcoholic Beverages in Childhood (in Per Cent)*

ITALIANS				ITALIAN AMERICANS				
Male	*Female*	*Total*		*Male*		*Female*		*Total*
				1st	2d+3d	1st	2d+3d	
(*N=125*)	(*N=122*)	(*N=247*)		(*N=28*)	(*N=81*)	(*N=44*)	(*N=98*)	(*N=251*)
1	0	0	Strong disapproval	0	4	2	4	3
2	2	2	Mild disapproval	4	4	0	7	4
1	1	1	Partial approval	0	0	0	0	0
17	24	20	Approval	89	79	89	75	81
70	68	68	Indifference	4	4	2	7	5
10	6	8	No information	4	10	7	6	7
101	*101*	*99*	*Totals*	*101*	*101*	*100*	*99*	*100*

toward the use of alcohol by the subjects when the latter were children. It is obvious that the majority of the fathers of the Italian subjects expressed indifference, while the majority of the fathers of the Italian-American subjects expressed unqualified approval.

Very nearly the same percentages of both fathers and mothers expressed the same opinions on the drinking of the subjects when they were children, on the drinking of the subjects when they were adults, and on the drinking of other adults. Among the parents of the Italian subjects, from 2 to 4 per cent expressed disapproval, 20 to 22 per cent expressed approval, and 64 to 70 per cent expressed indifference. Among the parents of the Italian Americans, from 1 to 4 per cent disapproved drinking by adults and 10 per cent disapproved drinking by children, 85 to 87 per cent approved drinking by adults and 78 to 79 per cent approved drinking by children, and 3 to 7 per cent expressed indifference.

No significant difference was apparent between the attitudes of the parents of male and those of female subjects.

Similar views were expressed by the subjects on the matter of their own drinking. Of the Italians, 1 per cent mildly disapproved, 15 per cent approved, and 80 per cent were indifferent. Of the Italian Americans, 2 per cent disapproved, 84 per cent approved without qualification, and 12 per cent expressed indifference. Essentially the same attitudes were expressed by the subjects toward drinking by other adults.

In the same way, the overwhelming majority of married Italian subjects expressed indifference to the drinking of their spouses, while the majority of married Italian Americans strongly approved. Similar opinions were presented by the spouses of the subjects.

So far as drinking by their own children was concerned, the great majority of Italian subjects and their spouses expressed indifference, while only a few voiced definite approval and practically none expressed disapproval. Among the Italian-American subjects and their spouses, however, approximately 6 per cent expressed indifference, 50 to 52 per cent expressed complete approval, 7 to 9 per cent expressed mild disapproval, and 4 to 5 per cent expressed strong disapproval. It appears that there is a mild trend among Italian Americans to disapprove of the use of alcoholic beverages by children. In all likelihood, however, this disapproval is far less prevalent than in other nationality groups.

The striking difference demonstrated here lies in the very high percentage of Italian subjects, both men and women, who are "indifferent" to the use of alcoholic beverages—who neither approve nor disapprove—and the high percentage of Italian Americans who strongly approve their use. It appears clear that, among the Italians, the answer "indifferent" really means "taken for granted." To them, when something is taken for granted, it does not have to be approved or strongly defended. In contrast, it appears that the Italian Americans—perhaps because they feel challenged by a new culture in which strong currents of thought and feeling oppose the use of alcoholic beverages—cannot hold a neutral, indifferent attitude. They have to be positive, and therefore they must approve.

In general, it may be concluded that very few subjects in the two groups even mildly disapproved of the use of alcoholic beverages. In addition, the overwhelming majority considered that alcohol—usually in the form of moderate amounts of wine—is not dangerous for children. This lack of fear has clearly survived immigration and the passing of generations.

Chapter 6

EXCESSIVE DRINKING

THE DEFINITION of intoxication is difficult to establish. The use of the term here is nontechnical and does not imply simply conditions arising from very high concentrations of alcohol in the blood. Such conditions occurred in the case of some of the subjects, but certainly not in most of them. What is meant by intoxication here is an ingestion of alcoholic beverages which led to some significant change in feeling, thinking or acting of the subjects—a change which, because of its nature, has not been forgotten even though it had no consequences, or only slight ones.

Patterns of Intoxication

The age at which the subjects reported having been first intoxicated is indicated in Table 44. The proportion of subjects who never experienced alcohol intoxication was substantially higher among the Italians than among the Italian Americans, and, as expected, higher among women than among men: 40 per cent of the men and 84 per cent of the women among the Italians, 43 per cent of the men and 57 per cent of the women among the first-generation Italian Americans, and only 16 per cent of the men and 49 per cent of the women among the second- and third-generation group.

It is interesting to note that a significant number of subjects—7 per cent of the Italians, 20 per cent of the first-generation Italian Americans, and 9 per cent of the second- and third-generation Italian Americans—recalled an episode of intoxication occurring before the age of 10. This fact must be considered within the frame of the definition of intoxication used here. According to the statements of the subjects, these early experiences occurred on the occasion of some party, festivity, religious holiday or the like, when the child—without consent of the parents—consumed wine in quantities not commensurate with his age.

The highest incidence of first episodes of intoxication occurred between the ages of 10 and 19. While first episodes also occurred between the ages of 20 and 29 for a considerable number of both Italians and Italian Americans, only a negligible number of subjects were over the age of 30 when they first experienced the effects of the excessive use of alcoholic beverages.

TABLE 44.—*Age (Years) at First Intoxication (in Per Cent)*

Italians				Italian Americans				
Male	*Female*	*Total*		*Male*		*Female*		*Total*
				1st	2d+3d	1st	2d+3d	
(*N*=*75*)	(*N*=*19*)	(*N*=*94*)		(*N*=*16*)	(*N*=*68*)	(*N*=*19*)	(*N*=*50*)	(*N*=*153*)
8	6	7	Under 10	13	10	26	8	12
50	22	45	10–19	31	62	16	32	43
38	50	40	20–29	44	24	16	44	31
3	17	5	30–39	0	0	11	12	5
0	0	0	40–49	6	1	5	4	3
0	0	0	50–59	6	0	11	0	2
1	6	2	No information	0	3	16	0	3
100	*101*	*99*	*Totals*	*100*	*100*	*101*	*100*	*99*

TABLE 45.—*Beverage Used in First Intoxication (in Per Cent)*

Italians				Italian Americans				
Male	*Female*	*Total*		*Male*		*Female*		*Total*
				1st	2d+3d	1st	2d+3d	
(*N*=*75*)	(*N*=*19*)	(*N*=*94*)		(*N*=*16*)	(*N*=*68*)	(*N*=*19*)	(*N*=*50*)	(*N*=*153*)
1	0	1	Beer	6	12	0	8	8
74	56	70	Wine	56	21	58	12	26
18	22	19	Distilled spirits	25	34	16	68	42
1	0	1	Aperitif	0	3	0	4	3
3	22	6	Combination	6	28	16	6	17
3	0	2	No information	6	3	10	2	4
100	*100*	*99*	*Totals*	*99*	*101*	*100*	*100*	*100*

As shown in Table 45, the beverage used by the Italian subjects at the time of the first intoxication was wine in 70 per cent of the cases, followed by distilled spirits in 19 per cent. Among the Italian Americans, distilled spirits was involved as the beverage in the first episode in 42 per cent of the cases, wine in 26 per cent, and beer in 8 per cent.

The total number of episodes of intoxication, as indicated in Table 46, was somewhat higher in the Italian-American group. It will be seen that 44 per cent of the Italians reported 3 or more such episodes during their lifetime, compared to 46 per cent of the first-generation Italian Americans and 48 per cent of the second- and third-generation group. The occurrence of 25 or more episodes was reported by 12 per cent of the Italians and 10 per cent of the Italian Americans.

The same data also demonstrate a markedly higher incidence among the Italian-American women. For instance, no Italian woman was intoxicated more than four times in her life, while this frequency was reported by 22 per cent of the Italian-American women. Four of the latter subjects listed more than 25 episodes of intoxication.

The type of alcoholic beverage most frequently used by the subjects when intoxicated is shown in Table 47. Wine was the beverage so used by the Italians, and distilled spirits by the Italian Americans.

The relationship between the beverage used and the frequency of episodes of intoxication is outstanding. The occurrence of such episodes is lowest among the Italians, who drink almost exclusively table wine. The frequency increases among the first-generation Italian Americans, who begin to drink more of other beverages. It is highest in the succeeding generations, who move still further away from the ancestral drinking customs and, presumably, the associated behaviors, attitudes and controls.

The companions with whom the subjects associated on the occasions when they became intoxicated are indicated in Table 48. This phase of drinking behavior was explored since the use of alcoholic beverages is often considered as an experience which favors social contacts. Of those Italians who reported some excessive use of alcohol, the majority stated that these episodes occurred in the presence of friends of both sexes. None reported such excessive drinking with friends of the opposite sex.

TABLE 46.—*Total Number of Episodes of Intoxication (in Per Cent)*

Italians Male	Italians Female	Italians Total		Italian Americans Male 1st	Italian Americans Male 2d+3d	Italian Americans Female 1st	Italian Americans Female 2d+3d	Italian Americans Total
(*N*=75)	(*N*=19)	(*N*=94)		(*N*=16)	(*N*=68)	(*N*=19)	(*N*=50)	(*N*=153)
31	63	37	1	38	31	63	46	41
19	16	18	2	6	12	0	16	11
20	21	20	3–4	31	19	11	18	19
9	0	7	5–9	6	10	5	12	10
7	0	5	10–14	0	9	0	0	4
0	0	0	15–19	6	0	5	2	2
0	0	0	20–24	6	1	0	0	1
15	0	12	25 or more	6	16	5	6	10
0	0	0	No information	0	1	10	0	2
101	*100*	*99*	*Totals*	*99*	*99*	*99*	*100*	*100*

TABLE 47.—*Beverage Most Frequently Used in Episodes of Intoxication (in Per Cent)*

Italians Male	Italians Female	Italians Total		Italian Americans Male 1st	Italian Americans Male 2d+3d	Italian Americans Female 1st	Italian Americans Female 2d+3d	Italian Americans Total
(*N*=75)	(*N*=19)	(*N*=94)		(*N*=16)	(*N*=68)	(*N*=19)	(*N*=50)	(*N*=153)
3	11	4	Beer	6	3	0	6	4
56	32	51	Wine	50	9	42	8	16
12	16	13	Distilled spirits	25	32	21	64	41
1	0	1	Aperitif	0	0	0	0	0
23	42	27	Combination	19	53	26	20	35
5	0	4	No information	0	3	11	2	3
100	*101*	*100*	*Totals*	*100*	*100*	*100*	*100*	*99*

TABLE 48.—*Companions during Episodes of Intoxication (in Per Cent)*

Italians: Male	Italians: Female	Italians: Total		Italian Americans: Male 1st	Italian Americans: Male 2d+3d	Italian Americans: Female 1st	Italian Americans: Female 2d+3d	Italian Americans: Total
(*N*=75)	(*N*=19)	(*N*=94)		(*N*=16)	(*N*=68)	(*N*=19)	(*N*=50)	(*N*=153)
0	0	0	No companions	0	4	5	2	3
79	53	73	Friends of both sexes	31	40	58	62	48
0	0	0	Friends of opposite sex	6	16	0	18	14
1	0	1	Friends of same sex	38	28	5	10	20
12	0	10	Friends in military service	19	6	0	0	5
4	37	11	Relatives	0	3	21	8	7
4	11	5	No information	6	3	11	0	3
100	*101*	*100*	*Totals*	*100*	*100*	*100*	*100*	*100*

TABLE 49.—*Occasion of Episodes of Intoxication (in Per Cent)*

Italians: Male	Italians: Female	Italians: Total		Italian Americans: Male 1st	Italian Americans: Male 2d+3d	Italian Americans: Female 1st	Italian Americans: Female 2d+3d	Italian Americans: Total
(*N*=75)	(*N*=19)	(*N*=94)		(*N*=16)	(*N*=68)	(*N*=19)	(*N*=50)	(*N*=153)
3	11	4	Childhood experiment	13	10	16	2	8
53	68	56	Parties, celebrations	50	65	58	88	70
13	0	11	In military service	19	7	0	0	5
0	0	0	Parties and in service	0	10	0	0	5
1	5	2	Other	6	3	16	8	7
29	16	27	No information	13	4	11	2	5
99	*100*	*100*	*Totals*	*101*	99	*101*	*100*	*100*

Among the Italian Americans who reported one or more episodes of intoxication, 31 per cent of the men and 58 per cent of the women in the first-generation group noted that these events occurred primarily in the company of friends of both sexes, as did 40 per cent of the men and 62 per cent of the women in the second- and third-generation group. It is noteworthy, however, that a significant proportion of the second- and third-generation Italian Americans reported that their companions during episodes of intoxication were friends of the opposite sex. Thus, there is little doubt that, when alone with members of the opposite sex, Italians seldom become intoxicated. The behavior of second- and third-generation Italian Americans is obviously different.

Of all subjects who reported the circumstances of episodes of intoxication, as shown in Table 49, approximately 60 per cent declared that these occurred at parties and celebrations, including weddings and Christmas and New Year's events. Only 4 per cent of the Italians who reported these details said the episodes occurred as the result of a childhood experiment, in comparison with 8 per cent of the Italian Americans. Only 2 per cent of these Italians and 7 per cent of the Italian Americans recalled that these experiences occurred during "other" occasions, such as during card games or on "dates."

Age and Frequency of Intoxication

Included in the Italian group were six men under the age of 20. Four of these had never been intoxicated, one reported being intoxicated once, and one from five to nine times. None of the five Italian women under the age of 20 had ever been intoxicated.

Among the Italian Americans, there were eight men and seven women—all second- and third-generation subjects—under the age of 20. All of the eight men and two of the seven women reported one or more experiences of intoxication.

The limited samples involved here do not permit any definite conclusions, but there may be a trend toward a higher incidence of intoxication at an earlier age in the Italian-American subjects.

Age at First Drink and Frequency of Intoxication

For the Italian men who were exposed to alcoholic beverages before reaching the age of 10 the numbers of episodes of intoxication were reported as follows: none, 36 per cent; 1–4, 50 per cent;

5–14, 8 per cent; and 15 or more, 6 per cent. For the men who were first exposed after the age of 10 the numbers of episodes were: none, 45 per cent; 1–4, 24 per cent; 5–14, 12 per cent; and 15 or more, 18 per cent.

The numbers of episodes for the Italian women who were exposed to alcohol before the age of 10 were as follows: none, 83 per cent; 1–4, 17 per cent. The numbers for the women who were exposed after the age of 10 were: none, 68 per cent; and 1 or 2, 32 per cent.

Among the Italian-American men exposed to alcohol before the age of 10 the numbers of episodes were: none, 25 per cent; 1–4, 50 per cent; 5–14, 12 per cent; and 15 or more, 13 per cent. For those first exposed after the age of 10 the numbers were: none, 24 per cent; 1–4, 48 per cent; 5–14, 16 per cent; and 15 or more, 12 per cent.

Among the Italian-American women the numbers of episodes for those exposed before the age of 10 were: none, 52 per cent; 1–4, 38 per cent; 5–14, 8 per cent; and 15 or more, 2 per cent. For those exposed after the age of 10 the numbers were: none, 46 per cent; 1–4, 46 per cent; 5–14, none; and 15 or more, 8 per cent.

A cautious evaluation of these percentages leads to the conclusion that among these subjects early exposure to alcoholic beverages does not seem to be linked with a larger number of episodes of intoxication.

Age at First Intoxication and Frequency of Intoxication

The age at first intoxication of those subjects who reported a total of 25 or more episodes of alcoholic intoxication was analyzed separately.

Of the 11 Italians who reported this number of episodes, only 1 was first intoxicated before the age of 10 and 6 were first intoxicated in their late teens.

Of the 2 first-generation Italian Americans who described 25 or more episodes, 1 was first intoxicated before the age of 10 and the other between the ages of 20 and 29.

Of the 14 second- and third-generation subjects with 25 or more episodes, only 2 were first intoxicated before they reached the age of 10.

It seems, thus, that among these subjects an isolated episode of intoxication before the age of 10 does not necessarily pave the way to frequent episodes of uncontrolled drinking in later life.

Distilled Spirits and Frequency of Intoxication

During the week of observation, only one Italian subject ingested distilled spirits in amounts representing from 6 to 9 per cent of the total caloric intake, and the other seven Italians who drank this beverage during the week ingested it in amounts representing 2 per cent or less of the caloric intake. Accordingly, members of the Italian group cannot be included in the present analysis.

Among the Italian Americans, 53 subjects ingested some distilled spirits, though none in amounts above 5 per cent of the total caloric intake. Of these subjects, however, 8 reported 25 or more episodes of intoxication during their lifetimes.

In addition to revealing a considerable number of episodes of intoxication among the subjects using distilled spirits, these data indicate that the information drawn from the dietary records, if evaluated individually, does not cast adequate light on the drinking habits of these individuals. Thus, it appears that in this group of Italian Americans excessive use of distilled spirits occurs only periodically and such an occurrence may be missed by an isolated study of a 7-day dietary diary.

Wine and Frequency of Intoxication

As in the case of distilled spirits, the use of wine as reported in the dietary diaries of the subjects was not evidently related to the total number of episodes of intoxication.

Of the Italian men, 13 drank no wine during the week of observation, yet 12 of them reported 1 or more episodes of intoxication during their lifetime.

Among the 9 subjects who reported 25 or more episodes, the amount of wine consumed during the week represented from 1 to 2 per cent of the total caloric intake for 1 subject, 3 to 5 per cent for 2, 6 to 9 per cent for 3, 15 to 19 per cent for 1, 20 to 24 per cent for 1, and 30 to 39 per cent for 1.

The largest numbers of episodes were, thus, reported alike by individuals who, during the week of observation, drank wine in very moderate amounts or in considerable amounts or who did not drink wine at all. In the case of the heavy drinker and the individual who has a proclivity toward the uncontrolled use of alcoholic beverages, it appears that the day-by-day pattern of drinking is not a mirror of events which are rather explosive in their onset and their manifestations.

Chapter 7

DISCUSSION: THE PREVENTION OF ALCOHOLISM

BECAUSE of their importance for both the physiological and psychological welfare of individuals and groups, the problems of alcohol have continued to absorb the interest of groups and populations all over the world. In this area, involving alcohol and alcoholism, the old controversy over the respective roles of heredity and environment—of "nature" and "nurture"—still rages, even though concealed under a different terminology. At the same time, an all-or-nothing attitude characterizes groups sometimes labeled "wets" and "drys" in their exclusive adherence to rigid and opposing doctrines.

In the controversy over alcohol and alcoholism, the strict opponents of all drinking have often insisted that availability of alcoholic beverages is the almost exclusive cause of the problems of alcohol. It cannot be denied that this availability and related social phenomena may play an important role in precipitating some of the problems of alcohol. It is highly doubtful, however, that this availability could be effectively prohibited. Moreover, even if these beverages could be made unobtainable, it is doubtful that this would be advisable where alcoholic beverages are valuable food items for many people.

Among the defenders of alcoholic beverages, too, there has been some inclination to take the narrow view that the problems of alcohol are represented exclusively by a limited number of individuals whose exceedingly deviant personality traits lead to excesses. The shift of emphasis from alcohol to the personality of the excessive drinker is largely justified with respect to alcoholism, but this does not mean that environmental conditions can be ignored.

Another class of theories that puts the problem essentially in a "nature" framework includes explanations of alcoholism as due to inborn physiological, biochemical, hormonal or metabolic traits (21, 29, 32). Unfortunately for such theories, the idea that alcoholism originates before or at birth has been surmised but not proved (7, 26). Accordingly, no serious investigator can endorse the proposal that merely some inborn inability to handle alcohol in a civilized way is the only difference between the 4½ million alcoholics in the U.S.A. (11) who should abstain entirely and the vast majority of adults who can drink moderately and without experiencing any difficulties.

In addition, overemphasis on inborn defects fails to offer solutions for problems connected with the use of alcoholic beverages —such as drunken driving or the release of sexual inhibitions under the influence of alcohol—which are not problems of alcoholism, and perhaps rarely concern the full-fledged alcoholics. There is ample evidence to support the claims that alcoholic beverages can be dangerous to persons other than true alcoholics.

Regrettably, the definition of an alcoholic is handicapped by the same difficulties which are involved when definitions are sought for any type of human behavior. To define means to limit and therefore to crystallize, but human behavior is dynamic, ever-changing and shifting, and can be described better than defined. Dynamic psychology is, to a large extent, incompatible with clear-cut definitions. Thus any statement defining 4 million or more alcoholics as radically different from all the other millions of adult Americans is open to serious challenge. The same traits which are typical of the alcoholic are often observed in individuals who either do not drink at all or, thus far, have been able to drink in moderation. These traits might remain latent for a time, flaring up only under exceptional circumstances, or they might remain latent forever.

A parallel situation exists in the area of sex. In the past, homosexuals were considered to be only those individuals who engaged in an act of sexual intercourse with a person of the same sex. When applied to sexual perversion, the modern and psychodynamically sound concept of latency leads to the conclusion that there are men and women who may never engage in active homosexual activities and yet constantly live under the painful pressure of homosexual strivings. In addition, more or less marked traits or seeds of homosexuality are observed in all human beings, and are interpreted as adult survivals of infantile and still unpolarized sexual drives. There is little doubt that, in certain circumstances, these latent homosexual traits—which ordinarily are kept under rigid control during the entire lifetime of an individual—can break through with great violence.

Here is obviously a situation in which "nature" and "nurture" interplay. The roles of those factors which are inborn or implanted very early in life are closely knit with those which result from later adult experiences. Clearly, then, it is a goal of a civilized society interested in the welfare of its citizens, in their emotional stability, and in the development of high ethical standards, to promote those environmental situations—the factors of "nurture"—which would favor heterosexual drives and thwart the homosexual tendencies.

The same holds true for the problems of alcohol. Besides the multitude of full-fledged alcoholics, there are certainly in this country millions of other adult individuals who harbor latent traits of addiction to alcohol. And just as the latent homosexual may become an active one as the result of a homosexual experience forced upon him, so the latent alcohol addict may respond to a suitable blood alcohol concentration—a concentration high enough to satisfy his drives—by setting in motion an addictive pattern of drinking.

There is no evidence, however, to support a belief that any experience with alcohol might cause such a flareup. Instead, it appears that the flareup may occur only if a sufficiently high blood alcohol concentration occurs in an individual at a time when the resistance of his central nervous system is low.

The Prevention of Alcoholism

The prevention of alcoholism, therefore, seems to require two courses of action:

1. Prevention of the development of those personality traits in the individual which are "addictive" in their nature, and which lead to latent predisposition to alcoholism.

2. Education inhibiting drinking practices which may lead to blood alcohol concentrations high enough to be appealing and pleasant to those individuals who may be harboring latent addictive traits.

When the prevention of latent "addictive" personality traits is under consideration, attention may well be focused particularly upon the experience of the Italians. It has been stated repeatedly that the incidence of alcoholism is low among them because of their way of drinking. In the eyes of the Italians, wine is a food. It is a liquid food as distinguished from solid food, but used in conjunction with the latter and consumed chiefly as a part of their meals.

In Italian nutrition, solid and liquid foods play complementary roles. Yet this does not entail such a blurring or erasing of distinctions as would imply that the individual had remained in or returned to the early, infantile stage of emotional development in which blurring of distinctions is natural.

In that early stage the infant can satisfy its hunger only within the frame of an intimate and mutually rewarding relationship with the mother or mother-substitute who feeds its body and at the same time favors its first social experiences. There is no distinction between hunger for food and hunger for love, or sociability; the two merge completely and are simultaneously fulfilled or simultaneously unfulfilled in the infant's relationship to its mother (17).

There is little doubt that the adequacy of this child–mother relationship deeply affects both the psychological growth and the social adjustment of the individual. While it is true that later events in life often minimize the importance of early experiences, these early events are never insignificant insofar as they served to demonstrate that the complete satisfaction of hunger could occur only through a secure social relationship. It is this kind of healthy relationship, marked in the infant by no clear distinctions between a hunger for food and a hunger for love, which leads to the development of a healthy, non-neurotic adult with healthy, unblurred distinctions—distinctions between what belongs to the body and what belongs to the mind, between the spiritual and the material.

On the other hand, the alcoholic or uncontrolled drinker appears to be emotionally unfit to accept such distinctions (14). His use of excessive amounts of alcohol seemingly represents an attempt to obtain the same type of blended, pleasurable experience which the infant obtains from milk. The alcoholic's striving for such blurred or blended pleasures in adulthood may result in large part from inadequate child–mother relationships in his infancy.

Mutually rewarding child–mother relationships, rediscovered by modern psychologists as essential to emotional stability, have long been an integral part of Italian and some other cultures. They have clearly played a role as one important factor in the prevention of alcohol addiction. They can play an equally important role in other cultures.

Alcoholism represents an unsuccessful attempt at free gratification of the individual's perverted instinctual needs. It is incompatible with the standards of a civilized society, and must be checked by the individual himself or, when he is unable to cope with the situation, by society. Further, society has the responsibility of protecting both the alcoholic and the latent alcoholic from the dangers inherent in their situations. It is in this area that "nurture" becomes of paramount importance.

So far as the obvious alcoholic is concerned, experience has proved time and again that only total and permanent abstinence from the use of alcoholic beverages can protect him.

For the person who may harbor latent traits of addiction to alcohol, the solution is by no means so simple or obvious. Presently available psychosocial techniques do not make it possible to predict accurately which latent addict will turn into the full-blown alcoholic. Thus, it might be suggested that total and permanent abstinence be urged—whether visibly essential or not—for all latent alcoholics. Such a proposal would appear to be somewhat impractical. Complete abstention from alcoholic beverages by large segments of the population of the Western World is far from a realistic possibility at present. The alternative is to utilize educational techniques to modify drinking behavior so that alcoholic beverages will be consumed under conditions least conducive to the unfolding of addictive traits. This clearly involves social approaches in an effort to shape customs and personality. The explosive dangers inherent in efforts of this kind are obvious, but they should not deter society from taking the necessary action.

Regardless of the type of alcoholic beverage, it is primarily the alcohol content which causes complications in the predisposed individual. For the alcoholic, an episode of intoxication is a lengthy and often fruitless attempt to achieve and then to maintain a "pleasure-yielding" concentration of alcohol in the blood (15). This pleasurable concentration cannot be described as a standard value since it varies from one individual to another, and from time to time in the same individual, though this concentration is fairly high. The variability results from the fact that the effects of alcohol are linked not only with alcohol concentrations in the blood stream but also with the state of the central nervous system, which mediates the effects of alcohol, as modified perhaps by the blood sugar level. Thus the establishment of an "addictive concentration" is the result of the interplay represented by the personality of the individual alcoholic considered as a composite of body and mind at the time of drinking, and the alcohol as well as other components in his internal environment.

The prevention of patent or full-fledged alcoholism should therefore be aided by two protective factors:

1. Those conditions which enhance the resistance of the central nervous system.
2. Restriction of drinking to amounts and patterns which lead to the lowest possible blood alcohol concentrations and are timed to occur when the resistance of the central nervous system is highest.

The Cocktail Hour

Against this background, it is interesting to consider the cocktail hour, a social institution which has crossed beyond the boundaries of the United States and is spreading widely abroad. The cocktail hour fulfills all the qualifications for favoring the development of latent addictive traits into obvious alcoholism.

Customarily scheduled late in the afternoon, the cocktail hour comes at a time when the individual's general resistance, and specifically the resistance of his central nervous system, are usually at their lowest ebb during the day. Fatigue is the theme of the hour.

This fatigue is partly the result of the day's work. It is, however, enhanced by dietary habits followed by many Americans—certainly by many of those who adhere to the cocktail custom. Their noontime meal is usually small, and sometimes is omitted.

In addition, the type of noon meal consumed by the majority of Americans includes only small amounts of slowly absorbable carbohydrates. Instead, it generally includes swiftly absorbable carbohydrates which lead to high blood sugar levels soon after lunch, followed by a reactive and marked hypoglycemia at the time of the cocktail hour. Thus the individual begins this hour in a state of general starvation plus a specific starvation for sugar—an internal environment which provides the central nervous system with little protection against the toxic effects of excessive amounts of alcohol.

During the cocktail hour itself, the individual drinks on an empty stomach. As a result, the alcohol is absorbed rapidly from the digestive tract, high blood alcohol levels are produced, and the alcohol is oxidized slowly.

Finally, as noted in the statements of many of the Italian Americans observed in this inquiry, participation in the cocktail hour is coupled with an attitude of drinking in a deliberate attempt to secure "sociability" or to achieve the "effects" of alcohol.

On both physiological and psychological grounds, it appears clear that the ingestion of alcoholic beverages within the frame of the cocktail hour is unhealthy. If a social institution had been consciously created to foster the development of latent alcohol-addictive traits, it is difficult to imagine how a more effective mechanism could have been devised.

The Safety Factor of Meals

In striking contrast, the ingestion of alcoholic beverages with meals provides the maximum protection to the individual and to the world in which he lives, and favors experiences which are beneficial. As a result of the presence of solid food in the stomach, the passage of alcohol into the bloodstream is delayed and the blood alcohol concentrations remain consistently lower than those noted when alcohol is ingested on an empty stomach (4).

Moreover, when alcohol is consumed on a full stomach, its rate of oxidation is relatively faster. The significance of this factor has only begun to be understood in very recent years. Oxidation means not only disposition of the alcohol and avoidance of potentially dangerous blood alcohol concentrations, but also rapid utilization of alcohol as a food and thereby a valuable contribution to the diet. It has been shown that these effects of a meal on the rate of alcohol oxidation persist for about 6 hours following ingestion of the solid food (27).

Further evidence of the advantages of using certain alcoholic beverages with meals has come from a study of the rate of synthesis of hippuric acid as an index of some liver functions (27). In that investigation, it was observed that even moderate amounts of alcoholic beverages—including wine—have a depressant action on hippuric acid synthesis if the beverages are consumed on an empty stomach. On the other hand, there is a distinct enhancement of hippuric acid synthesis—and presumably of liver function—when wine is ingested with a mixed meal.

It is not only for all these physiological reasons that the use of alcoholic beverages with meals provides the maximum safeguards. It is also because of the social setting involved, and the emotions connected with such a setting. If it is correct to state that behavior and misbehavior result to a large extent from early family experiences, then it appears obvious that the ingestion of alcoholic beverages within the frame of the healthy family provides the emotional background which can most effectively minimize dangers.

Chapter 8

SUMMARY AND CONCLUSIONS

AN INQUIRY was conducted on the eating and drinking habits of 247 Italians living in Italy and 251 Italian Americans living in the United States. The investigation included not only a study of the nutrition of these subjects—with special attention to their use of alcoholic beverages—but also an examination of their education, occupation, economic status, religious practices and attitudes, marital status, and general medical and psychiatric status. A number of individuals suffering from minor ailments were included in the study, but all cases with serious physical or mental illness were discarded. A detailed 7-day dietary record was obtained from each subject.

Although the two groups of subjects—the Italians and the Italian Americans—were considerably alike in many respects, they were not exactly comparable, and they do not necessarily portray the habits and attitudes of all Italians or of all Italian Americans. Nevertheless, many of the findings and comparisons appear to have some interest and significance, and may help in casting some light on the manner in which certain groups have long used alcoholic beverages safely and perhaps beneficially, while others have demonstrated a trend toward alcoholic excesses.

The major findings included the following:

1. In comparison with the Italian subjects, the Italian Americans were appreciably taller, more obese, more educated, and living on a higher economic standard. At the same time there was a slight movement toward marrying outside the church. None of the Italians but nearly 4 per cent of the Italian Americans were divorced.

2. The eating pattern among the Italians was more monotonous but more regular, while the Italian Americans demonstrated a tendency toward irregular, sporadic eating habits.

3. The majority of the Italian subjects were classified as "moderate eaters," while most of the Italian Americans were "heavy eaters."

4. Consumption of the main nutritional factors—proteins, fats and carbohydrates—was fairly adequate by both the Italian and Italian-

American groups. In general, the consumption of proteins and fats by the Italian Americans was relatively higher and the consumption of carbohydrates relatively lower. At the same time, it was observed that the carbohydrates obtained by the Italian subjects were from the more slowly absorbable carbohydrate foods, while the Italian Americans were more likely to indulge in the highly soluble and more quickly absorbable sugars. This last factor suggests that the dietary habits of the Italians may afford a greater protection against undesirable effects of alcoholic beverages.

5. Consumption of vitamins and minerals was likewise reasonably adequate in both groups, with the Italian Americans consuming relatively more calcium, phosphorus, iron, vitamin B_1, niacin, and Vitamin C.

6. Glucose tolerance tests resulted in the detection of 15 cases of hitherto unsuspected diabetes and 58 cases of borderline diabetes. Most of these subjects consumed relatively small quantities of alcoholic beverages.

7. The consumption of total fluids, alcoholic and nonalcoholic, including milk, "soft drinks," fruit juices, coffee and water, was strikingly higher in the Italian-American group. Only 1 per cent of the Italians but 38 per cent of the Italian Americans drank more than 400 ounces of fluids per week.

It may be noted here that the relatively low consumption of total fluids by the Italians is paralleled by a low incidence of alcoholism in this group, while the use of total fluids and the uncontrolled use of alcohol are both greater among the first-generation Italian Americans and greater still in the second- and third-generation group.

8. The consumption of total alcoholic beverages was higher among the Italians, and represented a substantially larger portion of the daily caloric intake. All alcoholic beverages together provided 10 per cent or more of the total caloric intake for 38 per cent of the men and 6 per cent of the women among the Italians, but for only 19 per cent of the men and 4 per cent of the women among the Italian Americans.

9. While wine remains a part of the normal daily diet of the Italians, its use has decreased noticeably among first-generation Italian Americans, and decreased even more in the second- and third-generation group. At the same time, among these Italian-

American subjects, there was an obvious increase in the use of beer and distilled spirits. Only 2 per cent of the Italians but 48 per cent of the Italian Americans reported the use of all four types of alcoholic beverages—beer, wine, aperitifs and distilled spirits.

10. Exposure to alcoholic beverages in early childhood was reported by most of the subjects, but the significance of such early drinking experiences was different in the two groups. Interpreted as part of a regular family, social or religious custom among the Italians, it represented a casual sip-taste experiment for the majority of the Italian Americans.

11. The Italians named "health" and "tradition" as major reasons for their present use of wine. In contrast, Italian Americans most often named "sociability" and "effect." The last reason was given by a substantially increased percentage of the Italian-American women.

12. While the majority of Italian Americans expressed strong approval of the use of alcoholic beverages by both children and adults, the majority of the Italians expressed only indifference. To the latter subjects it appears that such a use is taken for granted and accordingly needs no defense.

13. Most of the Italians but less than 10 per cent of the Italian Americans drank alcoholic beverages exclusively with meals. Combinations of drinking before, with, after and between meals were reported by 15 per cent of the Italians, 71 per cent of the first-generation Italian Americans, and 83 per cent of the second- and third-generation group.

14. Although the Italians regularly consumed alcohol in larger quantities, the occurrence of intoxication among this group was relatively uncommon. In striking contrast, the Italian Americans consumed less alcohol, but more of these subjects reported episodes of alcohol intoxication, and more of them reported the more frequent occurrence of such episodes. It appears that a decrease in the use of wine has been accompanied by an increase in the incidence of intoxication.

15. There seems to be little doubt that the custom of using alcoholic beverages separately from other food items—notably at the cocktail hour—is linked with a search for the psychological rather than the physiological effects of alcohol.

These findings seem to indicate that, for a variety of physiological and psychological reasons, the drinking behavior of the Italians in Italy provides a variety of protections against some dangerous effects of alcoholic beverages. When Italians are exposed to the American environment, however, the culturally determined protective patterns may be modified or lost. This has apparently occurred among the Italian Americans investigated here. The decline in the use of wine with meals and the increasing frequency of the use of alcoholic beverages other than wine before and between meals cannot fail to favor those conditions which are conducive to intoxication and the excessive use of alcohol.

Part II

Milk and Wine in Italy

BY

Pierpaolo Luzzatto-Fegiz, LL.D.

AND

Giorgio Lolli, M.D.

Chapter 9

THE PEOPLE AND THEIR DIETARY HABITS

AS a part of the survey of dietary practices of Italians in Italy and Americans of Italian extraction, carried out by cooperating staffs of the Istituto di Alimentazione e Dietologia in Rome and the Laboratory of Applied Biodynamics in New Haven, the Doxa Institute in Milan was requested to carry out an inquiry in a stratified sample of the adult population of Italy. In this survey, special attention was given to the consumption of milk and wine and to the attitudes of the population toward these important liquid constituents of the Italian dietary.

The Sample

A total of 1,453 adults were interviewed in this special study by a corps of 158 trained interviewers between 19 and 27 May 1954. The fundamental characteristics of the sample are described in the present section.

The sample was drawn from all persons aged 18 years and over and was composed of 48 per cent males and 52 per cent females. By age, they were classified as follows: 18–19 years, 4 per cent; 20–29, 24 per cent; 30–39, 25 per cent; 40–49, 19 per cent; 50–59, 14 per cent; and 60 or more, 14 per cent.

Unmarried subjects, both men and women, comprised 30 per cent of the sample, while 61 per cent were married and 9 per cent were widowed, separated or divorced.

By occupation, 4 per cent were listed as land owners or industrial executives, 18 per cent as farmers, 7 per cent as farmhands or other hired farm workers, 4 per cent as self-employed artisans, 7 per cent as skilled workers, 10 per cent as unskilled workers, domestics or heavy manual workers, 7 per cent as clerical employees or teachers, 1 per cent as minor executives or self-employed professionals, 31 per cent as housewives, 6 per cent as retired, 3 per cent as students, and 2 per cent as without occupation or unemployed.

While 9 per cent were described as wealthy, 43 per cent were classified as middle-class and 48 per cent as poor.

Most of the subjects lived in family units consisting of 3 to 5 members. The number of persons per family unit (including the subjects) was as follows: 1, 4 per cent; 2, 10 per cent; 3, 19 per cent; 4, 24 per cent; 5, 19 per cent; 6, 11 per cent; 7, 6 per cent; 8, 3 per cent; 9, 1 per cent; and 10 or more, 3 per cent.

The geographical distribution was 48 per cent in Northern Italy, 19 per cent in Central Italy, 23 per cent in Southern Italy, and 10 per cent in the Italian Islands.

Well over half lived in relatively small communities, with 30 per cent residing in communities of less than 5,000 population, 30 per cent in communities of 5,000 to 20,000, 14 per cent in communities of 20,000 to 50,000, 6 per cent in communities of 50,000 to 100,000, and 20 per cent in larger cities.

Asked to evaluate the apparent weight of the subjects, the interviewers classified 2 per cent of the men and 3 per cent of the women as "much overweight," 18 per cent of the men and 24 per cent of the women as "overweight," 53 per cent of the men and 46 per cent of the women as "normal," 23 per cent of the men and 22 per cent of the women as "underweight," and 4 per cent of the men and 5 per cent of the women as "much underweight."

As shown in Table 50, a trend toward underweight was noted in the younger subjects and a marked trend toward overweight in the older ones.

The Morning Meal

Breakfast was found to be a light meal for the overwhelming majority. Coffee was used alone by 35 per cent, and in the form of "cappuccino" (coffee with a little milk) or "caffelatte" (milk with a little coffee) by 42 per cent. Small amounts of bread or bread and butter were sometimes eaten with it. Milk was used alone by 13 per cent—10 to 11 per cent of the wealthy and middle-class groups and 15 per cent of the poorer subjects. Approximately 6 per cent reported eating nothing in the morning.

TABLE 50.—*Age in Relation to Apparent Body Weight (in Per Cent)*

	AGE CLASSES OF SUBJECTS				
	18–29	*30–39*	*40–49*	*50–59*	*60+*
Much overweight	1	1	3	4	6
Overweight	10	16	25	35	32
Normal weight	56	57	50	41	28
Underweight	29	23	18	18	23
Much underweight	4	3	4	2	11
Totals	*100*	*100*	*100*	*100*	*100*

Noon Versus Evening Meal

For 76 per cent of the sample—70 per cent of the men and 81 per cent of the women—the meal consumed at noontime was the largest and most important of the day.

It is hardly surprising that a relatively higher percentage of women considered the noon meal more important, since relatively more women were able to eat this meal at home.

Among the various age groups, relatively more of the oldest subjects—more than 85 per cent of those over the age of 60—described the noon meal as most important. This may be explained by the fact that the evening meal in Italy is usually eaten rather late, between 7 and 10 o'clock at night, and elderly people who retire soon afterward customarily prefer that this meal be light.

No marked differences in preference were noted according to geographic location, although it was observed that relatively fewer Southerners and Islanders than Northerners and Central Italians had their main meal at noon. The highest proportion of subjects who ate their main meal in the evening was observed in farmers living in very small municipalities and in industrial or white collar workers in the larger cities who customarily ate their noon meal at their place of employment.

While 84 to 85 per cent of the middle-class and wealthy ate their main meal at noon, this was reported by only 66 per cent of the poorer subjects in the sample. It is obvious that the underprivileged, partly because of their occupations, often found it impossible to have a regular noon meal.

Companionship at Meals

While the noon meal was generally eaten in surroundings dictated by employment or occupation, the evening meal was usually taken in company more closely representing the preferences of the subjects.

Only 10 per cent of the men and 8 per cent of the women customarily ate their evening meals alone, while 13 per cent of the men and 9 per cent of the women sometimes ate alone and sometimes ate with others, and 77 per cent of the men and 83 per cent of the women always or almost always shared their evening meals. There is little doubt that this pattern is common in western civilizations. In such cultures, it appears that there is almost always a drive toward socialized eating experiences, and that only emotionally disturbed individuals are definitely repelled by the idea of sharing meals with other people.

This repulsion to eating in company has been noted in some extremely disturbed food addicts whose eating experiences bear a connotation of almost sexual intimacy—a connotation which forbids any sharing. Typical of such individuals is a 42-year-old woman, 5 ft. in height and weighing 280 lbs., who declared that, so far as she could remember, she had never eaten a meal in the presence of friends, relatives, or anyone else. Her statement was corroborated by her mother and other members of her family.[1]

Eating the evening meal always or almost always alone was reported by 19 per cent of the unmarried men but only 13 per cent of the unmarried women. In the Italian culture, it appears that either the family gives more supervision to the single woman than to the single man, or that this supervision is sought more by the single woman.

The custom of eating the evening meal in solitude was observed most frequently among widows and widowers and more frequently among the latter.

Further inquiry revealed that members of the Italian families talked with no evident inhibitions at meal time, discussing whatever was of direct interest to one or more members of the group. Similarly, outbursts of anger occurred rather frequently at mealtimes, regardless of the age, sex, marital status, geographical area or social class of the subjects. It appears that such emotional discharges did not affect family cohesion unfavorably but rather represented outlets for pent-up emotions whose unrelieved pressure might otherwise have had more serious consequences.

Eating Between Meals

As expected from the earlier nutritional inquiry on Italians and Italian Americans, it was found that the great majority of the Italians here—76 per cent of the men and 67 per cent of the women—did not eat between meals. It is interesting to note that the percentage is lower for the women even though food is presumably more accessible to them at home.

Among those who did eat between meals, the preferred food items were salami or sausage with bread; bread only; cheese; and fresh fruit.

[1] Lolli, G. [Unpublished observations.]

Eating between meals was reported by 44 per cent of those under 30 years of age, 25 per cent of those between 30 and 49, and less than 20 per cent of those over the age of 50.

Contrary to expectation, it was noted that social status apparently had little effect on the percentage of those who habitually ate between meals, although the foods consumed were somewhat different. Among the poorer subjects who reported between-meal eating, the most commonly used foods were salami and sausage with bread, bread only, or cheese. Among the middle-class and wealthy subjects, the preferred foods for this purpose were salami and sausage with bread, cakes, pies, candy, and fresh fruit.

Drinking Between Meals

The beverages consumed between meals are shown in Table 51. It is obvious that drinking between meals is more common than eating between meals, and that beverages are used in such fashion more frequently by men than by women.

The beverage most commonly used was wine, followed by coffee or "cappuccino," and water. So far as wine is concerned, it is evident that when taken with meals this beverage is used almost equally by men and women. Taken between meals, however, wine appears to be more a man's beverage, being ingested by 40 per cent of the Italian men and only 7 per cent of the women. Milk was consumed between meals by only a small portion of the sample.

TABLE 51.—*Beverages Consumed Between Meals (in Per Cent)*

	Male	*Female*	*Total*
Wine	40	7	23
Coffee or "cappuccino"[1]	16	16	16
Water	15	17	16
Tea	2	8	5
Aperitifs[2]	5	3	4
Beer	6	1	3
Milk	2	5	4
Soft drinks[3]	6	5	6
Mineral waters	0	2	1
Liqueurs & "Grappa"	2	1	1
"What I find at home"	0	2	1
None	31	50	41
Totals[4]	*125*	*117*	*121*

[1] "Cappuccino" is coffee with a little milk.
[2] Including vermouth and dessert wines.
[3] Including orangeade, lemonade, cola drinks, quinine water and other nonalcoholic beverages.
[4] Totals over 100 per cent because of multiple responses.

TABLE 52.—*Beverages Consumed Between Meals, by Social Class (in Per Cent)*

	Wealthy	*Middle*	*Poor*
Wine	10	20	28
Coffee or "cappuccino"	26	19	11
Water	8	14	20
Tea	14	7	2
Aperitifs	11	5	1
Beer	5	4	3
Milk	8	4	2
Soft drinks	9	8	3
Mineral waters	2	2	0
Liqueurs & "Grappa"	3	1	1
"What I find at home"	1	1	1
None	34	39	43
Totals[1]	*131*	*124*	*115*

[1] Totals over 100 per cent because of multiple responses.

Age seemed to have little bearing on the consumption of beverages between meals, except perhaps in the case of wine. This beverage was ingested by 17 per cent of those between the ages of 18 and 29, 29 per cent of those between 30 and 39, 20 per cent of those between 40 and 49, 27 per cent of those between 50 and 59, and 24 per cent of those aged 60 or over.

The use of wine between meals was reported by 28 per cent in Northern and Central Italy, respectively, 15 per cent in Southern Italy, and 12 per cent in the Islands. Coffee in one form or another was used by 9 per cent in the Islands and by 16 or 17 per cent in other areas. Water was used by 25 per cent in the Islands and by 15 to 17 per cent of those living elsewhere. Milk was used by 6 per cent in Northern Italy and by 1 or 2 per cent in the other areas.

Striking differences in the use of beverages between meals were noted in the different social groups, as shown in Table 52. It is obvious that drinking between meals was most common among the wealthy and least frequent among the poorer subjects. Wine was seldom used between meals by the wealthy, occasionally by middle-class subjects, and most frequently by poorer individuals. Coffee and "cappuccino" were used most frequently by the wealthy, as were the relatively expensive aperitifs and liqueurs. Water, the cheapest beverage available, was understandably used most frequently by the poorer subjects. Tea, used mostly by the wealthy,

TABLE 53.—*Beverages Consumed Between Meals, by Occupation (in Per Cent)*

	Executives[1]	Farmers	Farmhands	Artisans	Skilled Workers	Unskilled Workers	White-Collar Workers	Housewives	Others[2]
Wine	15	54	51	13	26	26	3	6	18
Coffee or "cappuccino"	25	10	5	20	21	14	36	17	15
Water	12	22	21	7	15	19	7	19	6
Tea	8	1	1	2	1	1	8	9	6
Aperitifs	18	1	0	6	4	1	17	2	1
Beer	4	5	5	6	6	5	5	0	1
Milk	6	2	1	0	2	1	4	5	9
Soft drinks	16	1	3	9	5	5	12	6	3
Mineral waters	0	1	1	2	1	1	0	1	1
Liqueurs & "Grappa"	4	2	0	0	2	0	1	1	1
"What I find at home"	4	1	1	0	0	0	0	1	0
None	25	27	31	54	39	41	37	50	49
Totals[3]	*137*	*127*	*120*	*119*	*122*	*114*	*130*	*117*	*110*

[1] Executives, property owners, professional workers.
[2] Retired workers, students, unemployed.
[3] Totals over 100 per cent because of multiple responses.

still appears to be considered a foreign drink, with little appeal to middle-class or poor groups.

Equally significant differences were noted in the use of beverages between meals according to occupations, as shown in Table 53. The highest percentage of individuals who drank nothing was observed among artisans and housewives, the lowest among executives, farmers and farmhands. Wine was used most frequently by farmers —both owners and farmhands—and least frequently by white-collar workers. The most frequent use of coffee occurred among white-collar workers and the most frequent use of water among farmers.

These data clearly indicate that those engaged in heavy manual labor were inclined to use wine between meals, while those engaged in sedentary activities were more likely to use coffee. It is interesting to note that the same occupational groups which most frequently consumed wine were also the groups which most frequently used water. Multiple factors were presumably involved. In all likelihood, the need to replace water lost through heavy physical labor accounted at least in part for its consumption by manual workers,

TABLE 54.—*Attitudes of Subjects Toward Size of Own Meals, by Age Class and Sex (in Per Cent)*

Attitudes, Males	*18–29*	*30–39*	*40–49*	*50–59*	*60+*	*Total*
Too much	5	7	4	3	5	5
Plenty, but not too much	31	19	25	27	13	23
Just right	48	59	62	48	43	53
Little, but enough for me	9	13	5	16	28	13
Too little	7	2	4	6	11	6
Totals	*100*	*100*	*100*	*100*	*100*	*100*
Attitudes, Females						
Too much	6	5	9	9	3	7
Plenty, but not too much	17	12	8	9	9	12
Just right	51	59	54	57	46	53
Little, but enough for me	18	19	22	18	35	21
Too little	8	5	7	7	7	7
Totals	*100*	*100*	*100*	*100*	*100*	*100*

while the same workers also used wine because of its energy-yielding qualities. The stimulating effect of coffee on the central nervous system may have accounted for its preference by those who lead a sedentary life.

Quantity of Diets

The opinions expressed by the subjects concerning the amount of their own daily food intake are summarized in Table 54. This information does not necessarily indicate that the respondents are good judges of their diet but it appears to provide valuable clues to their nutritional attitudes.

It seems significant that all subjects had some opinion about their diets, and that only a small proportion—11 per cent of the men and 14 per cent of the women—felt they were eating substantially too much or too little.

More than half of both the men and the women described their food intake as "just right." This appears to be a rather high proportion, especially if it is considered that the nutritional pattern of each individual represents the grouping and interacting of a variety of psychological, physiological and social factors. It is possible that, of those individuals who claimed that they ate "just right," a considerable number more or less consciously attempted to conceal deviations of nutritional habits about which they experienced conscious or unconscious guilt. The emotions linked with eating habits are fundamental. Deviations in such habits are constantly associated with emotional problems, often guilt-laden, and therefore likely to be concealed (16).

It will also be noted that many more men than women feel that they eat "plenty, but not too much," while more women than men report that they eat "little, but enough for me."

Of the subjects who were rated overweight by the interviewers, only 9 per cent stated that they ate too much. This low incidence supports the view that guilt-laden nutritional habits are often concealed. An additional 20 per cent of these apparently overweight individuals declared that they ate "plenty, but not too much," while 17 per cent said they ate "little, but enough for me" and 6 per cent said they ate "too little." These last answers may be completely realistic for some of the overweight subjects. There is no doubt that an overweight person ate too much in his past life, but it is not necessarily true that he eats more than the average at the time his weight has stabilized.

Of those who were rated normal in weight, 6 per cent thought they ate "too much," 17 per cent "plenty, but not too much," 60 per cent "just right," 14 per cent "little, but enough for me," and 3 per cent thought they ate "too little."

Of those who were rated underweight, 3 per cent said they ate "too much," 15 per cent "plenty, but not too much," 45 per cent "just right," 25 per cent "little, but enough for me," and 12 per cent thought they ate "too little."

The reasons for overeating as offered by those who claimed they ate too much are shown in Table 55. It is not surprising that the majority of these subjects stated that they overate because they felt hungry. A distinction must be drawn, however, between hunger and the physiological needs of the individual. Although it is true that hunger is an instinct that develops in order to satisfy some

TABLE 55.—*Reasons for Overeating Given by Subjects Who Ate "Too Much" (in Per Cent)*

	Male	*Female*	*Total*
Hunger	56	56	55
Gluttony	14	12	13
Desire to gain weight	6	4	5
Cannot control eating	8	10	9
For health	8	12	11
Other reasons	0	4	2
"I do not know"	8	2	5
Totals	*100*	*100*	*100*

TABLE 56.—*Reasons for Undereating Given by Subjects Who Ate "Too Little" (in Per Cent)*

	Male	*Female*	*Total*
Financial	37	36	37
Lack of appetite	34	21	27
Health	18	25	22
Fear of gaining weight	3	12	8
Other reasons	3	4	3
"I do not know"	5	2	3
Totals	*100*	*100*	*100*

definite physiological need and to contribute to the maintenance of the internal environment of the individual, it is also true that, because hunger is closely linked with psychological and social factors, these factors may increase the urge to eat even when real physiological needs are lacking.

In Table 56 is a summary of the reasons for undereating as given by those who claimed they ate too little. More than 85 per cent cited financial factors, lack of appetite, or health. Diet control to prevent gain in weight was mentioned by only a few of the women—most of these between the ages of 18 and 29—and by even fewer men. This difference in male and female attitudes could probably be found in other western cultures, suggesting that concern over weight gain may be motivated more by standards of beauty or fashion than by fears of any illness which might be related to obesity.

On the other hand, when all subjects were questioned on the relative desirability of different weight deviations, approximately four times as many preferred being moderately underweight to moderately overweight.

Quality of Diets

Of the entire sample, 79 per cent gave the opinion that their diet was nutritionally satisfactory to both their tastes and their needs, 15 per cent described their diet as unsatisfactory, and 6 per cent expressed uncertainty.

In terms of ideal nutrition, these diets may or may not have been adequate, but they were obviously acceptable to most of the Italians, enabling them to live in reasonable comfort and to perform useful activities. This general attitude obviously fits into the basic philosophy of the majority of Italians who, as a result of deeply ingrained cultural attitudes, have learned not to ask too much of life and to be content with what life offers.

Greater satisfaction with their diets was expressed by Northern and Central Italians than by those living in other areas of the country. This conforms to the belief that the diet in Northern and Central Italy is generally more adequate than that in Southern Italy or the Italian Islands.

While 87 per cent of those in the wealthy and middle classes considered their diets satisfactory, only 69 per cent of the poorer subjects expressed such an opinion. In all likelihood, the reported inadequacy of diets by the wealthy is either imaginary or the result of physical or emotional disorders which interfere with proper nutrition.

The reasons given by those who expressed dissatisfaction with their diets are presented in Table 57. Most of these subjects stressed their inadequate protein consumption, the lack of nourishing food, and the fact that their diet did not appeal to their tastes. It is clear that relatively more men than women believe their protein intake is inadequate. This seems to be based on the concept, unproved but widely accepted, that men have some natural, physiological need for a higher intake of calories and a correspondingly higher intake of proteins.

Among the middle-class subjects in this group of dissatisfied individuals, 32 per cent claimed they were unable to eat according to their tastes, 17 per cent declared they did not eat enough meat, 17 per cent complained their diet included food items of limited nutritional value, and 12 per cent said they were forced to remain

TABLE 57.—*Reasons for Inadequate Diet Given by Subjects Who Reported Diet Unsatisfactory (in Per Cent)*

	Male	*Female*	*Total*
Not enough meat	41	29	35
Not enough fresh fruit	5	10	8
Not enough eggs	5	4	5
Not enough sugar & sweets	4	6	5
Not enough seafood	7	5	6
"I do not eat what I like"	16	16	16
Lack of nourishing foods	27	24	25
Diet monotonous	4	4	4
Limited financial means	5	11	8
Diet required by illness	6	8	7
Other reasons	3	4	3
"I do not know"	1	3	2
Totals[1]	*124*	*124*	*124*

[1] Totals over 100 per cent because of multiple responses.

TABLE 58.—*Reasons for Inadequate Diet Given by Subjects Who Reported Diet Unsatisfactory, by Apparent Body Weight of Subjects (in Per Cent)*

	Much Over-weight	*Over-weight*	*Normal*	*Under-weight*	*Much Under-weight*
Not enough meat	29	35	39	36	14
Not enough fresh fruit	14	5	11	6	5
Not enough eggs	14	0	5	8	0
Not enough sugar & sweets	0	5	4	6	5
Not enough seafood	14	3	5	9	4
"I do not eat what I like"	43	14	17	11	23
Lack of nourishing foods	14	27	17	31	45
Diet monotonous	14	0	5	5	0
Limited financial means	0	5	8	9	14
Diet required by illness	0	14	7	5	4
Other reasons	0	8	4	0	4
"I do not know"	14	0	2	2	0
Totals[1]	*156*	*116*	*124*	*128*	*118*

[1] Totals over 100 per cent because of multiple responses.

on an unsatisfactory diet because of illness. Among the poorer subjects, 41 per cent blamed a lack of sufficient meat, 28 per cent reported use of food items of limited nutritional value, and 11 per cent claimed that limited financial means were responsible. The proportion of the wealthy in this group was too small to permit further analysis.

Table 58 presents an analysis of the reasons given for inadequate diet according to the apparent weight of the subjects. From the totals alone, it is obvious that the overweight subjects gave the greatest number of reasons, expressing dissatisfaction with their diet on many different grounds.

Few subjects in any of these groups pointed to a lack of sugar or sweets in general.

It is apparent that a sizable percentage of even the overweight individuals expressed the opinion that their diet included food items of limited nutritional value. This should not be surprising. Overweight men and women, feeling guilt over their predicament, may consciously or unconsciously try to prove to themselves or to the outside world that their diet is not responsible for their obesity.

Chapter 10

ATTITUDES TOWARD MILK AND WINE

IN this special investigation on a stratified sample of Italian adults, major attention was focused on the significance of milk and wine: first on the beliefs and attitudes expressed by the subjects and then on the manner in which they put their beliefs into actual practice.

The opinions expressed by the subjects on the values of the two beverages are presented in the following sections.

Appreciation of Milk

At the outset, 71 per cent of the sample (62 per cent of the men and 78 per cent of the women) expressed a liking for milk. Most of these were individuals who used this beverage as part of their breakfast.

In contrast, 19 per cent (24 per cent of the men and 16 per cent of the women) stated that they disliked milk, while 10 per cent (14 per cent of the men and 6 per cent of the women) reported that they were indifferent or "did not like milk much."

This appreciation of milk was not significantly affected by age, geographical location, social class, or size of community in which the subjects lived. Accordingly, it appears that these attitudes are implanted early and deeply in the personality of Italians.

Value of Milk with Breakfast

Three-quarters of the sample, as shown in Table 59, expressed the belief that it is healthy to drink milk at breakfast. This appears to be a relatively low value. In many other societies of the Western world, it is probable that larger portions of the population would endorse this use.

No significant differences were found according to age, geographical location or social class.

Among those who claimed that the breakfast use of milk is unhealthy, the reasons for such an opinion included the beliefs that milk is difficult to digest, it is "heavy," it causes stomach acidity, it is fattening, it contains microbes, it depresses the appetite, and it is "bad" in the cities. Some subjects claimed that wine is preferable to milk.

TABLE 59.—*Attitudes on Healthfulness of Milk with Breakfast (in Per Cent)*

Attitude	*Male*	*Female*	*Total*
Healthy	70	81	75
Unhealthy	5	3	4
Neither	10	7	9
"I do not know"	15	9	12
Totals	*100*	*100*	*100*

Value of Milk and Wine with Lunch and Dinner

A comparison of the attitudes on the use of milk and of wine with the noon and evening meals is given in Table 60.

While three-quarters of the sample considered it desirable to use milk with breakfast, less than one-third expressed such an attitude in respect to the noon or evening meal. In striking contrast, more than three-quarters endorsed the use of wine with these major meals.

The major support for the use of milk with lunch or dinner came from wealthy respondents, of whom 38 per cent described this use as healthy, in contrast to only 25 per cent of the poor and 31 per cent of the middle-class groups.

Whereas the use of milk was favored by more women than men, the use of wine was endorsed by more men than women. In the Italian culture, it appears that milk may have a "childish" and perhaps a "feminine" connotation, while wine is more "masculine."

Similarly, it is obvious that the use of wine with meals is a subject which offers few chances for dissension. Only 1 per cent claimed that this was unhealthy, in contrast to 12 per cent who opposed the use of milk with major meals. While 8 per cent were unable to formulate any opinion about wine, 26 per cent were uncertain about the value of milk.

No large differences on the value of wine with meals were noted

TABLE 60.—*Attitudes on Healthfulness of Milk and Wine with Lunch and Dinner (in Per Cent)*

	MILK			WINE		
Attitude	*Male*	*Female*	*Total*	*Male*	*Female*	*Total*
Healthy	25	32	29	86	72	79
Unhealthy	12	12	12	1	1	1
Neither	35	31	33	8	16	12
"I do not know"	28	25	26	5	11	8
Totals	*100*	*100*	*100*	*100*	*100*	*100*

TABLE 61.—*Reasons Cited for Believing Use of Milk with Meals Unhealthy (in Per Cent)*

	Male	*Female*	*Total*
Favors indigestion, is heavy	27	22	24
Not compatible with other foods	16	21	18
Causes diarrhea, stomach ache, etc.	14	17	16
"I prefer wine"	21	10	15
Causes acidity	8	13	11
Milk is complete food in itself	7	5	6
Other reasons	2	9	6
"I do not know"; no answer	8	7	8
Totals[1]	*103*	*104*	*104*

[1] Totals over 100 per cent because of multiple responses.

according to age or geographical location. When occupations were analyzed, it was found that the greatest support for wine came from farmers, skilled and unskilled workers, property owners, executives and professional men and women, while the least came from self-employed artisans, white-collar workers and housewives.

Table 61 summarizes the reasons given by those who declared the use of milk with meals to be unhealthy. It appears significant that 21 per cent of the men and 10 per cent of the women declared that milk was unhealthy on the grounds that they preferred wine. The same view was expressed by 8 per cent of the wealthy, 12 per cent of the middle-class and 20 per cent of the poor. Among the wealthy, the main reasons for opposing the use of milk with meals were based on the indigestibility or "heaviness" of this beverage, and the belief that milk is a complete food in itself. The majority of the middle-class and of the poor opposed milk on the grounds that it favors indigestion, is "heavy," is not compatible with other foods, or causes diarrhea, stomach ache, acidity and similar symptoms.

Those few subjects—1 per cent of the sample—who believed the use of wine with meals to be unhealthy gave the following reasons: alcohol is harmful; wine is ethyl alcohol; wine is unhealthy because of the presence of ethyl alcohol; "I am a teetotaler;" or wine hampers the digestive processes, raises blood pressure, is an irritant, makes people sleepy and decreases efficiency, stimulates the central nervous system, overworks the kidneys, does not mix with food, and is constantly harmful to elderly people. Only one of the 1,453 respondents declared that "people acquire the habit of drinking and turn into drunkards." Clearly, the possibility that the use of

TABLE 62.—*Beliefs Concerning Amounts of Wine which Can be Consumed Daily Without Harm by Heavy and Light Workers (in Per Cent)*

Amount (liters)	HEAVY WORKERS *Male*	HEAVY WORKERS *Female*	HEAVY WORKERS *Total*	LIGHT WORKERS *Male*	LIGHT WORKERS *Female*	LIGHT WORKERS *Total*
¼	0	2	1	5	13	9
½	7	15	11	31	41	37
¾	2	5	4	7	6	6
1	29	34	32	39	25	32
1½	20	13	16	8	5	6
2	26	18	22	6	2	4
2 & more	14	5	9	1	0	1
"Don't know"	2	8	5	3	8	5
Totals	*100*	*100*	*100*	*100*	*100*	*100*

wine with meals might favor the onset of alcoholism is alien to the thoughts and feelings of Italians.

Recommended Safe Amounts of Wine

Further evidence of the widespread acceptance of the safety of wine is contained in the opinions expressed on the quantities of this beverage which may be consumed without harm.

Table 62 shows the quantities which the respondents estimated could be taken safely by adults doing heavy and light work, respectively. For individuals engaged in heavy manual labor, it was thought that an average of 1.4 liters of wine could be consumed daily in safety, and nearly half of the respondents set the figure at 1.5 liters or more. For adults doing light work, it was suggested that 0.8 liter of wine could be consumed each day without harm.

It may be noted that 1 liter of the common Italian wine corresponds to between 3 and 3.5 oz. of absolute alcohol or 6 to 7 oz. of whisky.

In general, men were less conservative in approving the use of larger volumes of wine for both heavy and light workers. As will be noted later, the actual wine consumption reported by the subjects is significantly less than the amounts they rated as harmless.

Implicit in the different estimates here is the concept that wine is an energy-yielding food and is utilized as such by workers—a concept common also in France (12).

Recommended Uses of Milk

Although the use of milk with lunch and dinner was considered a healthy habit for all people—children and adults alike—by only

TABLE 63.—*Attitudes on Use of Large Amounts of Milk by Children and the Elderly (in Per Cent)*

	USE BY CHILDREN			USE BY ELDERLY		
Attitude	*Male*	*Female*	*Total*	*Male*	*Female*	*Total*
Healthy	86	91	88	56	67	62
Unhealthy	3	2	3	10	8	9
"Don't know"; no answer	11	7	9	34	25	29
Totals	*100*	*100*	*100*	*100*	*100*	*100*

29 per cent of the sample, this use was more strongly endorsed for children and for elderly people. A summary of the views in these areas is given in Table 63.

Women were somewhat more aware than men of the nutritional value of milk for children, for this use in large amounts was recommended by 86 per cent of the men and 91 per cent of the women. Large quantities of milk for children were similarly approved by 91 per cent of the wealthy and middle-class and by 86 per cent of the poor subjects, and by 84 per cent of the Southern Italians and 88 to 90 per cent of those in other areas of the country.

As in the case of children, the use of milk in large amounts by elderly people was favored more by women than by men. It appears at least doubtful that whole milk, with its high fat content, is a safe food for middle-aged and elderly people. It is possible that skimmed, fat-free milk would be endorsed with fewer misgivings.

The use of milk by the elderly was endorsed more strongly by the wealthy and middle-class subjects than by the poor, and more strongly by those living in the Italian Islands than by those in other areas.

General Evaluation of Milk

In order to ascertain the over-all attitudes of the subjects toward milk, they were requested to give true-or-false assessments to a number of statements commonly made to describe the advantages of this beverage. Their opinions are shown in Table 64.

Approximately two-thirds agreed that milk is a complete food, that it is particularly suitable for weak persons, and relatively inexpensive when its nutritional values are considered. About one-quarter of the subjects confessed their ignorance on these points. Only one-quarter agreed that milk can provide strength to athletes, while two-thirds stated that they did not know.

Relatively more women than men were convinced that milk is

TABLE 64.—*Reactions to Common Statements on the Advantages of Milk (in Per Cent)*

Statement	*True*	*False*	*Don't Know*	*Total*
Milk is one of the most complete foods	71	4	25	100
Milk is a food suited to weak persons	67	8	25	100
Considering its nutritional value, milk is one of the cheapest foods	66	11	23	100
Milk gives strength to athletes	23	9	68	100

a complete food and one particularly useful to weak individuals, while more men than women—especially more young men—expressed the belief that milk gives strength to athletes. Relatively more wealthy and middle-class subjects rated milk highly as a complete food and as relatively inexpensive, while more middle-class and poor subjects agreed that it was especially useful for weak persons.

General Evaluation of Wine

The subjects were similarly asked to consider the accuracy of statements commonly used to describe the advantages of wine. Their views are given in Table 65.

With 61 per cent indicating that wine is nourishing and 79 per cent that wine gives strength, it is obvious that the majority had some awareness of the energy-yielding qualities of wine. Only 15 per cent, however, believed that wine is more nourishing than milk while 44 per cent rejected this statement.

It is important to note here that, in equal volumes, the typical wine used by the Italians yields approximately the same number of calories as does milk. The yield of calories is naturally not the sole indication of the nutritional value of a food. Because of its multiple constituents, milk is a more complete food than wine. It remains to

TABLE 65.—*Reactions to Common Statements on the Advantages of Wine (in Per Cent)*

Statement	*True*	*False*	*Don't Know*	*Total*
Wine is nourishing	61	14	25	100
Wine gives strength	79	7	14	100
Wine is more nourishing than milk	15	44	41	100
Good wine is harmless, even in considerable amounts	26	46	28	100

be proved, however, that adults living on a balanced diet have any need for large amounts of milk.

The statement that wine is nourishing was considered true by 68 per cent of the men and 55 per cent of the women, and by more elderly than young subjects. The statement that wine gives strength was endorsed by 85 per cent of the men and 74 per cent of the women, regardless of age. The statement that wine is more nourishing than milk was approved by 21 per cent of the men and 9 per cent of the women but was rejected by nearly half the subjects. This last statement was endorsed more frequently by older than by younger men, and more frequently by younger than older women. It is noteworthy that while 26 per cent thought wine harmless even in "considerable" amounts, 46 per cent rejected this statement and 28 per cent were uncertain.

Chapter 11

USES OF MILK AND WINE

THE preceding chapter was devoted to the various attitudes and opinions expressed by the subjects on the desirability and values of milk and wine. Information on the actual uses of these two beverages is presented in the present chapter.

Early Use of Milk

As noted elsewhere (17), experiences connected with breast feeding in infancy may be of fundamental value to the adult-to-be in the prevention of later physical illness and emotional maladjustment, including excessive drinking and alcoholism.

In the present stratified sample, 73 per cent reported having been breast fed by mother, 6 per cent by a wet nurse, and 6 per cent by a combination of breast and artificial feeding. In addition, 10 per cent did not know about this early experience, and it is probable that some of them were breast fed. Thus not less than 85 per cent and possibly more than 90 per cent of these subjects were breast fed in infancy at least in part, acquiring through the mother's milk not only the necessary nutrients but also the security and love which appear to be indispensable for proper adult adjustment.

It seems to be highly significant that so many subjects were aware that they had been breast fed. This awareness, of course, did not depend on the personal recollection of the individuals but reflected facts discussed in the presence of the growing child or disclosed to him by mother, father or other close relatives. There were obviously few adult inhibitions concerning this experience.

The highest percentage of breast feeding by the mother was reported by middle-class subjects and the lowest by the wealthy, while the highest percentage of individuals fed by a wet nurse was found among the wealthy.

Lack of information was reported by 16 per cent of the men and 5 per cent of the women, and by 5 per cent of the wealthy subjects, 8 per cent of the middle-class group, and 13 per cent of the poor.

The use of milk after weaning is indicated in Table 66. Consumption of this beverage seems to decrease progressively from the age of 10 to the age of 20.

TABLE 66.—*Use of Milk During Childhood Periods, as Reported by Subjects (in Per Cent)*

	Much	*Little*	*None*	*Don't Know*	*Total*
Immediately after weaning	39	14	3	44	100
Up to 10 years	43	30	7	20	100
At 10–15 years	31	43	16	10	100
At 15–20 years	22	45	25	8	100

Early Use of Wine

As shown in Table 67, at least half the men and one-third of the women began the use of wine before reaching the age of 15. This refers not to the first exposure to wine but to the beginning of its regular use. In the case of small children, this beverage was given in infinitesimal amounts and usually diluted with water.

No significant regional differences were observed for this early experience.

Use of Milk and Wine with Lunch and Dinner

A marked discrepancy between attitudes and actual practices was noted when the respondents described their own use of milk and wine.

As was shown in Table 60, 29 per cent expressed the opinion that it is healthy to drink milk with the noon and evening meals, and 79 per cent that it is healthy to drink wine. So far as their own drinking habits were concerned, however, only 3 per cent regularly used milk while 81 per cent used wine with these main meals.

The primary reasons given for their actions by those who did not use milk with lunch and dinner were "I don't like it"; "I don't like it while I eat"; "I'm not in the habit of using milk"; or simply,

TABLE 67.—*Age at Which Regular Use of Wine Began (in Per Cent)*

Age (years)	*Male*	*Female*	*Total*
1–4	11	7	9
5–9	18	10	14
10–14	23	17	20
15–19	16	12	14
20–24	6	9	7
25 and more	1	1	1
Don't drink wine	4	15	10
Don't remember; no answer	21	29	25
Totals	*100*	*100*	*100*

"I prefer wine." In addition, some subjects claimed that milk is "heavy" and hard to digest.

Use of Milk and Wine Between Meals

Only 2 per cent of the subjects reported the daily use of milk between meals, 2 per cent used it "often," 24 per cent used it "sometimes," and 72 per cent (79 per cent of the men and 65 per cent of the women) never used it in this fashion.

The use of wine between meals was reported by 23 per cent (40 per cent of the men and 7 per cent of the women). The wine was usually taken in small quantities. This use was reported most frequently by farm owners and farmhands and least frequently by white-collar workers and housewives.

The major reasons given by those who did not use milk between meals were "I don't like it"; "I'm not in the habit of using it"; "it is harmful, difficult to digest, or heavy"; or "I prefer wine."

Amounts of Milk and Wine Consumed

The quantities of milk used are indicated in Table 68, which shows weekly consumption of whole milk alone or mixed with coffee or cocoa. The preference of adult Italians for milk mixed with other beverages is evident.

Only 2 per cent drank whole milk in amounts of 5 or more liters a week, approximately a quart a day.

The average amount of wine consumed daily with each main meal—lunch and dinner—is shown in liters in Table 69.

TABLE 68.—*Amounts of Milk, Alone and Mixed with Coffee or Cocoa, Used Weekly (in Per Cent)*

Amount (liters)	*Milk Alone*	*Milk with Coffee or Cocoa*
½	5	6
1	8	11
1½	4	8
2	9	12
2½	1	2
3	5	5
3½	2	2
4	2	2
4½–5	1	1
5 & more	2	1
None; no answer	61	50
Totals	*100*	*100*

TABLE 69.—*Amounts of Wine Used Daily With Each Main Meal and Between Meals (in Per Cent)*

Amount	WITH MEALS			BETWEEN MEALS		
(liters)	*Male*	*Female*	*Total*	*Male*	*Female*	*Total*
Less than ⅛	7	33	20	8	6	7
⅛–¼	24	30	27	12	4	8
¼–½	36	7	21	15	1	8
½–¾	16	2	9	7	0	3
¾–1	6	0	3	7	0	3
1 & more	1	0	1	3	0	2
None	10	28	19	48	89	69
Totals	*100*	*100*	*100*	*100*	*100*	*100*

The mean average consumption with each meal was 0.25 l. for all subjects, drinkers and nondrinkers, in the group—0.36 for the men and 0.14 for the women. For those subjects who reported drinking wine with meals, the average was 0.31–0.40 l. for the men and 0.19 for the women. As might be expected, the consumption with meals was related to the body weight of the subjects; the mean average consumption with each major meal was 0.33 l. for those wine-users who were apparently overweight, 0.30 for those who were normal, and 0.29 for those who were underweight. The largest consumption of wine with lunch and dinner was observed among farmers and farmhands, the smallest among white-collar workers and housewives.

Information on the average amounts of wine used daily between meals is also presented in Table 69. Of those who drank wine at such periods, two-thirds of the men and all of the women used less than 0.5 l. per day in total.[1]

[1] For additional data on the use of wine in Italy see Luzzatto-Fegiz (22).

Chapter 12

DISCUSSION AND CONCLUSIONS

THE ATTITUDES toward milk and wine, and the actual consumption of these beverages, may together help to illuminate some of the major factors which—at least in the Italian population—have served to prevent alcoholic excesses and alcohol addiction.

The appreciation of milk is especially pertinent. Milk is the first food to which the newborn child is exposed, a food which supplies not only physical nourishment but also the protection and the security of a mother's love. It provides the child with mixed or blended or confused pleasures of body and mind (17). Most of the healthy, fundamental emotions which lead to adequate growth and social adjustment of the individual are linked with the experiences involving the use of milk by the infant, and to the resultant relationships between mother and child.

To the Italians in the present sample, believed typical of the Italian population, milk is the ideal food for the infant, especially if it is obtained through the overwhelmingly prevalent experience of breast-feeding.

In adult life, however, it is obvious that the use of milk is viewed quite differently. It is not considered outstandingly healthy in the opinion of large segments of the Italians, and it is not widely used by them.

There are many emotional and cultural reasons which may help explain this adult attitude. Milk-borne epidemics of typhoid fever were the source of great fears in the past. Milk is considered to be "baby food" by very large segments of the population. Since lukewarm milk may evoke overly vivid memories of childhood experiences, it is possible that some opposition to the adult use of milk in Italy is partly a consequence of inadequate refrigeration. It might well be that the more favorable attitudes of the North American population toward the use of milk are dependent in part on better refrigeration facilities and on the availability of a cold, odorless milk which can satisfy nutritional needs and infantile emotional longings without being identified as "baby food."

Whatever the reasons, it is clear that the vast majority of Italians are not convinced of the value of milk as a complete, healthy or necessary food for the adult. On the other hand, the vast majority of these people are convinced that it is healthy for adults to drink wine with meals, and their beliefs are matched by their habits. They ingest large amounts of wine with their main meals—a physiological and psychological setting in which the individual can best utilize the assets of wine and simultaneously neutralize any of its possible liabilities.

No emphasis is placed by the Italians on any "psychological" or "escape-providing" qualities of wine, and only a single person among the 1,453 subjects expressed fear that the use of wine might lead to alcoholism.

In short, the majority of Italians demonstrate their conviction that milk is for consumption by the healthy child and wine is for consumption—with meals—by the healthy adult.

The attitudes and actions of an alcoholic are strikingly different. To a certain extent, alcohol represents to the alcoholic what milk represents to the infant (14). Alcohol gives to the adult alcoholic a combination of physiological and psychological satisfactions which, in many ways, seem comparable to the gratifications supplied by milk to the infant. As an adult, the alcoholic seems to be seeking experiences which he missed—or thinks he missed—in his childhood. During the brief and painful periods of awareness in the final stages of alcoholism the alcoholic seems to be restlessly searching for alcohol in the same way the newborn infant searches for milk.

This confusion is obviously uncommon among Italians, for the incidence of alcoholism among these people—notwithstanding their large use of wine—is very low.

Though the low incidence of alcoholism in Italy is matched by a low adult consumption of milk, and there is a conversely high incidence of alcoholism in some countries where the adult consumption of milk is high, any notion that it is this use of milk which primarily determines the rate of alcoholism would be absurd and totally without foundation. It would be equally absurd, however, to hope that alcoholism might be alleviated or prevented by such simple devices as increased consumption of milk by adults. Only identification of the underlying causes of alcoholism and their alleviation can be effective in this problem of mental health.

Summary and Conclusions

An inquiry on broad nutritional habits, with particular emphasis on attitudes toward milk and wine and the actual uses of these important beverages, was conducted in a stratified sample of adult Italians in Italy.

1. The least important meal of the day was breakfast, while the noon meal was considered the largest and most important.

2. Eating in solitude was relatively uncommon. Most subjects ate their evening meal with family members or other companions.

3. Irregular or sporadic eating patterns were infrequent, and eating between meals was uncommon.

4. In general, most of the subjects appeared satisfied with the amount of their diets.

5. Most subjects appeared satisfied with the quality of their diets. The greatest deficiency was reported as a lack of protein.

6. More than 70 per cent stated that they like milk; 75 per cent thought it healthy to drink milk with breakfast; but less than 30 per cent believed it healthy to drink milk with lunch or dinner. Approximately 12 per cent declared it is unhealthy to drink milk with meals.

7. The use of milk with meals was more favored for children and the elderly.

8. Milk was rated higher by women than by men, and by wealthy and middle-class respondents than by the poor.

9. Milk was considered the ideal food for the infant. More than 85 per cent of the sample had been breast fed in infancy, and could discuss this experience with few or no adult inhibitions. The subjects continued to use milk but in steadily decreasing amounts from early childhood to adolescence and early adulthood. At the same time, there was presumably a parallel decrease in the emotional attachments to milk which expressed the psychological rather than the physiological needs of the individual.

10. During those youthful periods, the use of wine with meals became increasingly frequent. More than half the men and one-third

of the women reported beginning the regular use of wine before reaching the age of 15.

11. As adults, 29 per cent of the subjects considered it healthy to drink milk with lunch or dinner, but only 3 per cent actually did so. In contrast, 79 per cent expressed the opinion that it is healthy to drink wine with these meals and 81 per cent actually did so.

12. While 79 per cent said it is healthy to drink wine with meals, only 1 per cent claimed it is unhealthy and only 1 person out of 1,453 expressed fear that the drinking of wine could lead to alcoholism.

13. The average estimate by the subjects was that 1.4 liters of wine could be ingested each day by heavy workers and 0.8 l. by light workers without harm. The actual intake of the subjects was substantially less, averaging 0.31 l. with each major meal, or 0.62 l. per day, for all those who drank wine.

14. The largest quantities of wine were approved for use by those engaged in heavy labor, indicating widespread acceptance of wine as an important energy-yielding food. The nourishing values of wine were accepted by more men than women, and by more elderly than young respondents.

15. Between meals, milk was consumed daily or often by 4 per cent and wine by 23 per cent, including 40 per cent of the men and 7 per cent of the women. Wine was used most frequently between meals by those engaged in heavy physical labor.

It appears, therefore, that Italians consider milk the ideal food during the individual's growth. A physiologically and psychologically proper administration of milk to the infant, especially through breast feeding, prepares him for a physiologically and psychologically proper administration of wine, in moderate amounts and with solid food, when he becomes an adult.

Since the Italian adults ingest only small amounts of milk, with or between meals, the low rate of alcoholism in Italy cannot be attributed simply to milk consumption.

This survey yielded no evidence that a high adult consumption of milk would either favor or prevent alcohol addiction.

Bibliography

1. BACON, S. D. Sociology and the Problems of Alcohol. Foundations for a Sociological Study of Drinking Behavior. New Haven; Hillhouse Press; 1944. Also in: Quart. J. Stud. Alc. **4:** 402–445, 1943.
2. BARNETT, M. L. Alcoholism in the Cantonese of New York City; an anthropological study. In: DIETHELM, O., ed. Etiology of Chronic Alcoholism; pp. 179–227. Springfield, Ill.; Thomas; 1955.
3. HAGGARD, H. W. and GREENBERG, L. A. The effects of alcohol as influenced by blood sugar. Science **85:** 608–609, 1937.
4. HAGGARD, H. W., GREENBERG, L. A. and LOLLI, G. The absorption of alcohol; with special reference to its influence on the concentration of alcohol appearing in the blood. Quart. J. Stud. Alc. **1:** 684–726, 1941.
5. HAGGARD, H. W. and JELLINEK, E. M. Alcohol Explored. Garden City, N.Y.; Doubleday; 1942.
6. JELLINEK, E. M. An outline of basic policies for a research program on problems of alcohol. Quart. J. Stud. Alc. **3:** 103–124, 1942.
7. JELLINEK, E. M. Heredity of the alcoholic. In: Alcohol, Science and Society; Lecture 9, pp. 105–114. New Haven; Quarterly Journal of Studies on Alcohol; 1945.
8. JELLINEK, E. M. Estimate of number of alcoholics and rates of alcoholics per 100,000 adult population (20 years and older) for certain countries. In: EXPERT COMMITTEE ON MENTAL HEALTH. Report on the First Session of the Alcoholism Subcommittee. World Hlth Org. Techn. Rep. Ser., No. 42. Geneva; 1951.
9. JELLINEK, E. M. Distribution of alcohol consumption and of calories derived from alcohol in various selected populations. Proc. Nutr. Soc. **14:** 93–97, 1955.
10. KELLER, M. and EFRON, V. Illustrative Statistics on Alcohol Problems, 1955. *Pt. I.* The Extent of Drinking; Table 12. New Haven; Journal of Studies on Alcohol, Inc.; 1955.
11. KELLER, M. and EFRON, V. The prevalence of alcoholism. Quart. J. Stud. Alc. **16:** 619–644, 1955.
12. LEBRETON, E. and TRÉMOLIÈRES, J. Part de l'alcool dans le dépense calorique. Proc. Nutr. Soc. **14:** 97–102, 1955.
13. LISANSKY, E. S., GOLDER, G., and LOLLI, G. Relationship of personality adjustment to eating and drinking patterns in a group of Italian Americans. Quart. J. Stud. Alc. **15:** 545–561, 1954.
14. LOLLI, G. The addictive drinker. Quart. J. Stud. Alc. **10:** 404–414, 1949.
15. LOLLI, G. Alcoholism as a medical problem. Bull. N.Y. Acad. Med. **31:** 876–885, 1955.

16. Lolli, G. Centers for research on nutritional habits and for the prevention and correction of their deviations. Quart. J. Stud. Alc. **16:** 393–396, 1955.
17. Lolli, G. Alcoholism as a disorder of the love disposition. Quart. J. Stud. Alc. **17:** 96–107, 1956.
18. Lolli, G., Serianni, E., Banissoni, F., Golder, G., Mariani, A., McCarthy, R. G. and Toner, M. The use of wine and other alcoholic beverages by a group of Italians and Americans of Italian extraction. Quart. J. Stud. Alc. **13:** 27–48, 1952.
19. Lolli, G., Serianni, E., Golder, G., Balboni, C. and Mariani, A. Further observations on the use of wine and other alcoholic beverages by Italians and Americans of Italian extraction. Quart. J. Stud. Alc. **14:** 395–405, 1953.
20. Lolli, G., Serianni, E., Golder, G., Mariani, A. and Toner, M. Relationships between intake of carbohydrate-rich foods and intake of wine and other alcoholic beverages. A study among Italians and Americans of Italian extraction. Quart. J. Stud. Alc. **13:** 401–420, 1952.
21. Lovell, H. W. and Tintera, J. W. Hypoadrenocorticism in alcoholism and drug addiction. Geriatrics **6:** 1–11, 1951.
22. Luzzatto-Fegiz, P. Gli Italiani e il Vino. Milano; Edizione Doxa; 1952.
23. Malraux, A. Replies to 13 Questions. Partisan Rev. **22:** 157–170, (Spring) 1955.
24. National Research Council, Food and Nutrition Board. Recommended Dietary Allowances. Revised, 1948. National Research Council Reprint and Circular Series, No. 129. Washington; Oct. 1948.
25. National Research Council, Food and Nutrition Board, Committee on Nutrition Surveys. Nutrition Surveys, Their Techniques and Value. National Research Council Bulletin, No. 117. Washington; May 1949.
26. Roe, A., Burks, B. and Mittelmann, B. Adult Adjustment of Foster Children of Alcoholic and Psychotic Parentage and the Influence of the Foster Home. (Memoirs of the Section on Alcohol Studies, Yale University, No. 3.) New Haven; Quarterly Journal of Studies on Alcohol; 1945.
27. Serianni, E., Cannizzaro, M. and Mariani, A. Blood alcohol concentrations resulting from wine drinking timed according to the dietary habits of Italians. Quart. J. Stud. Alc. **14:** 165–173, 1953.
28. Skolnick, J. H. A study of the relation of ethnic background to arrests for inebriety. Quart. J. Stud. Alc. **15:** 622–630, 1954.
29. Smith, J. J. The endocrine basis and hormonal therapy of alcoholism. N.Y. St. J. Med. **50:** 1704–1706, 1711–1715, 1950.
30. Snyder, C. R. Alcohol and the Jews. A Cultural Study of Drinking and Sobriety. (Monographs of the Yale Center of Alcohol Studies,

No. 1.) New Haven, Publications Division of the Yale Center of Alcohol Studies; and Glencoe, Ill., Free Press; 1958.

31. Williams, P. and Straus, R. Drinking patterns of Italians in New Haven. Quart. J. Stud. Alc. **11:** 51–91, 250–308, 452–483, 586–629, 1950.

32. Williams, R. J. The etiology of alcoholism: A working hypothesis involving the interplay of hereditary and environmental factors. Quart. J. Stud. Alc. **7:** 567–587, 1947.

Index